try it!

STYLE YOUR HAIR

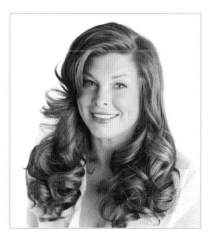

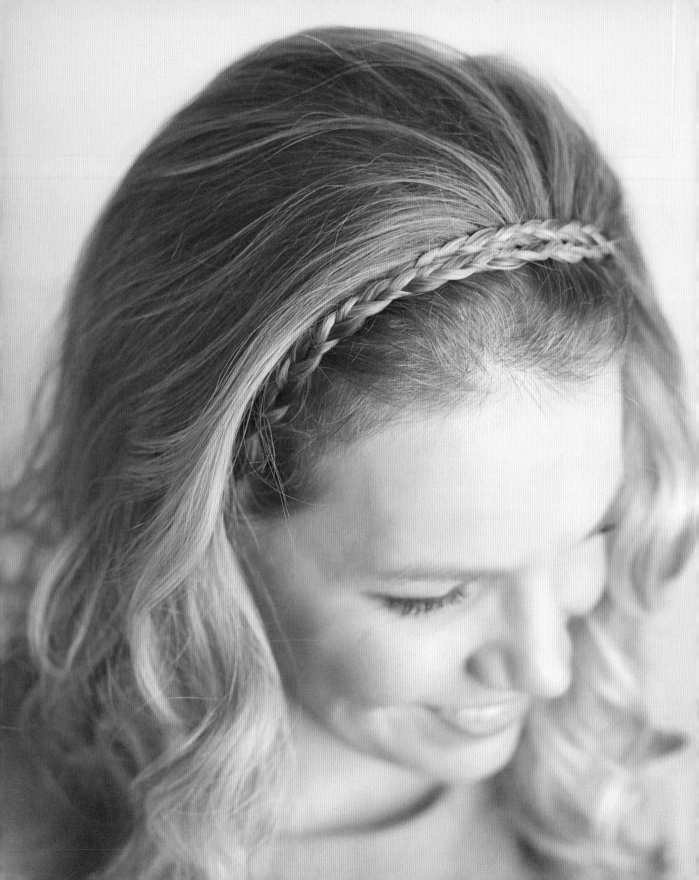

try it!

STYLE YOUR HAIR

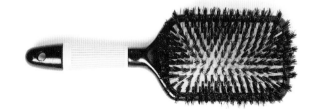

Contents

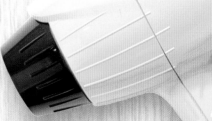

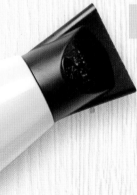

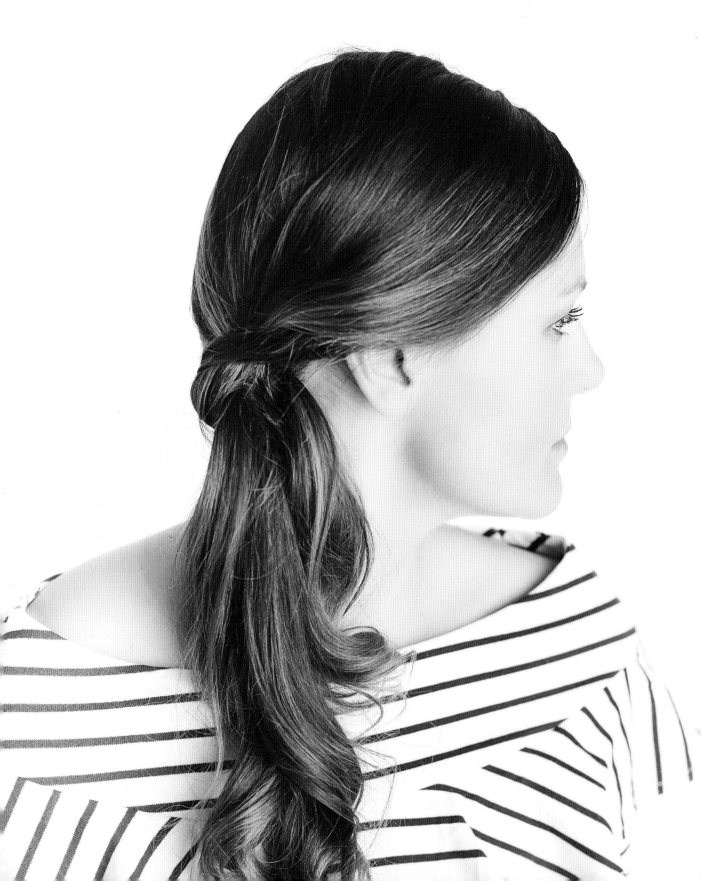

Introduction

I'm instantly taken back to my first trip to the salon with my mother. Maybe you have a similar childhood memory of that occasion. I can remember the entire atmosphere: the smells, the sounds, the products, the stylist. But most of all, I remember my mother's demeanour when we left the salon. She seemed happy and confident with her new look. She also seemed to have an extra bounce in her step that afternoon. Something about that day resonated with me, and I couldn't wait to go back and get my hair styled, so I could feel just as beautiful as my mother did. Looking back now, as someone in the role of hairstylist, it's my goal to make everyone who sits in my chair or reads this book look and feel their absolute best.

Even if you've never picked up curling tongs, a round brush, or hair grips, I assure you that you can create a variety of hairstyles, whatever your hair length, with the help of this book. In it, I explain the best ways to prep your hair before you begin a style and explain which tools and styling products to use and when. Then the fun begins, as I walk you, step by step, through each of the styles and show you how to create salon-worthy finished looks at home – complete with tips on fun ways to accessorize your new hairdo.

Learning to style your own hair shouldn't be frustrating – it should be rewarding. Take your time and follow the easy, how-to steps laid out here. It may take you a few tries to master the basic steps, but once you've got to grips with these essentials, you'll be styling your hair into that party-perfect ponytail, French plait, or chignon, with no effort at all.

If you come across something you're unsure of, simply turn back to the hairstyling basics pages or to the glossary for additional assistance.

One of the most confusing aspects of hairstyling is knowing which type of product to use on your hair, and how and when to apply it. Product manufacturers produce collections specific to each hair type and to benefit every texture, so that's a good place to start. It's best to work with what you have naturally and gently coax it to behave how you want it to. In addition to product distribution and usage, certain styling techniques also help in creating specific looks. All of this and more is covered in the following pages.

When you're ready for a bit more of a challenge, I've included formal styles that take you from birthday party to red carpet, as well as some looks for younger family members. None of these styles should be intimidating. Simply follow the text instructions and the helpful photos, and you'll soon discover that these styles are really quite manageable.

Read this book cover to cover, or pick and choose the parts that interest you most. However you use it, you're sure to gain a wide variety of techniques and skills to build your hairstyling knowledge with the help of this guide. Everything I've included has been helpful to me along the way, and I hope the same is true for you as you discover how fun and rewarding it can be to style your own hair. You'll save money, gain tons of confidence in your abilities to style your own hair, and look and feel beautiful – as if you've just stepped out of the salon.

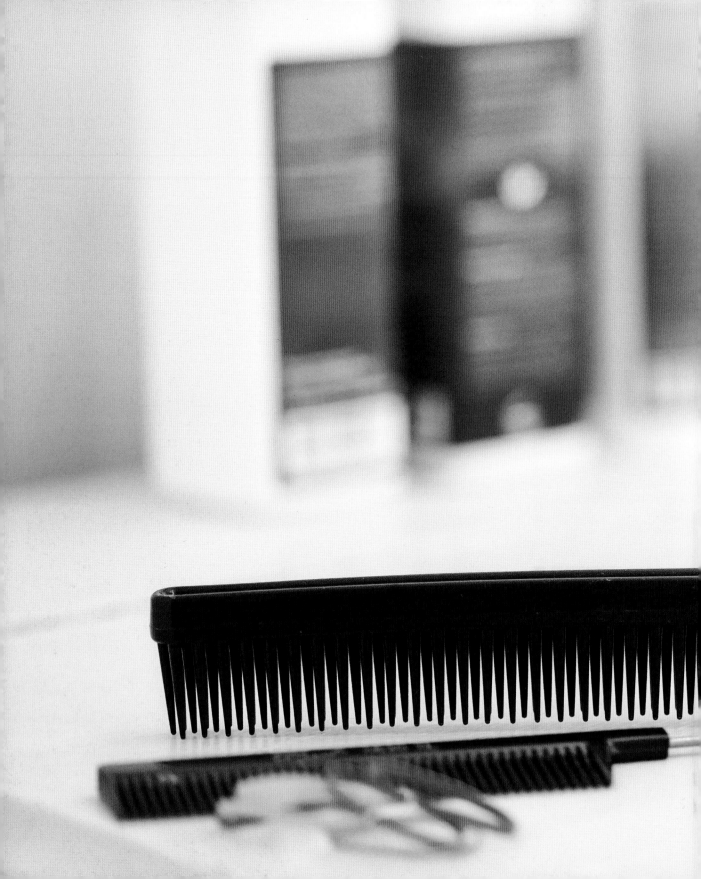

Tools of the
Trade

Hair-styling tools and gadgets may come and go, but there are some basic, classic tools that never go out of fashion. Once you have learned their purpose and how to use them correctly, you won't want to be without them. In this section, you meet the styling products, tools, and aids recommended for the hairstyles in this book. Some you might already own; others might be new to you. But in every case, you'll find handy tips and tricks on how and when to use them.

If you've ever seen a fantastic hairstyle and wondered how the look was achieved, you can stop wondering after reading this section. The descriptions clearly explain what each tool or product does, and how it can help you achieve the style you want. These are everyday styling aids found at your local chemist or beauty store, and they are easy to use with a few simple techniques and a little practice.

Styling Products

With so many styling products available at your hair salon, on chemist and supermarket shelves, and online, trying to decide which shampoo, conditioner, and other styling products will suit your hair can be confusing. But rather than buying a generic, one-size-fits-all product, it's worth taking some time to learn about the various styling products available, so you can choose one that is best for your specific hair type.

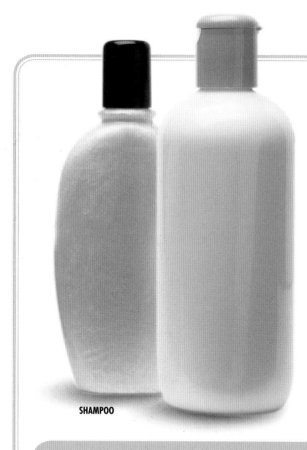

SHAMPOO

Shampoo

Shampoo manufacturers produce myriad options for every type and texture of hair. Here are a few types you might see:

VOLUMIZING SHAMPOO

This lightweight shampoo is meant to give limp locks some lift. It's usually transparent in colour, and should give your hair a weightless feel, without stripping the hair of its natural oils. You can use this type of shampoo to get rid of the silicone build-up that can sometimes occur with frequent use of serums and other styling products.

THICKENING SHAMPOO

This shampoo is best for those whose hair is thinning or who have very fine hair to begin with. It often contains an exfoliating ingredient to unclog follicles and give your strands the best possible chance of growth, as well as thickness-boosting ingredients.

Gently does it

If you wash your hair every day, choose a gentle shampoo that is labelled as suitable for frequent washing. This will help prevent your hair from drying out.

HYDRATING SHAMPOO

This shampoo is normally a bit heavier, and designed for dry or dull hair. If you have fine hair, you should generally avoid hydrating or moisturizing shampoos, since these can weigh down your hair. Medium to thick and coarse hair types benefit most from this type of shampoo.

REPAIRING SHAMPOO

This shampoo helps improve the texture and appearance of hair that has been damaged by heat or chemical treatments. It can also help reduce future breakage.

DRY SHAMPOO

This shampoo is every girl's best friend and a quick and easy hairstyle extender. By using this oil-absorbant spray, you can freshen up a two- or three-day-old style. You also can add texture to your hair by applying dry shampoo to your roots and using a backcombing comb. This is a great tip for formal styles, too.

Conditioner

After shampooing your hair clean, conditioner is the first product you should put back in. Conditioners come in a variety of types for different purposes:

VOLUMIZING CONDITIONER

This weightless formula is meant to soften your tresses, without leaving behind any residue that might weigh them down. Fine to medium hair types benefit most from a lightweight volumizing conditioner.

HYDRATING CONDITIONER

If you have curly locks, or are prone to frizz, this is the conditioner for you. Hydrating conditioners often contain natural oils, such as olive or argan oil.

REPAIRING CONDITIONER

This product often contains a protein or keratin treatment to help strengthen weak or damaged hair. If you regularly colour your hair, or use hot tools frequently, aim to use this type of conditioner at least once a week.

Mix and match

Manufacturers may prefer you to use matching shampoo and conditioner, but there's no reason you can't mix different brands, choosing whichever products you like best.

THICKENING CONDITIONER

This conditioner is meant to be used alongside thickening shampoo, and helps add natural volume to limp or lifeless strands. It softens the hair without weighing it down.

LEAVE-IN CONDITIONER

This conditioner comes as either a cream or a spray. Most leave-in treatments contain a moisture-retention ingredient, as well as ingredients to help protect your hair. Leave-in conditioners can offer different levels of moisture, depending on your hair type. Many also add shine to your locks.

Styling

This category of products is the largest – and often the most confusing. The lifters, lotions, powders, and other potions in this section all have specific uses and can smooth, tame, boost, or add bounce to your hairstyle:

ROOT LIFTER

This booster gives your hair a lift at the roots, especially in the crown area. Opt for a root lifter that's not too sticky to touch, and that leaves your hair soft.

SCULPTING LOTION

This light-hold formula gives hair hold without weighing it down. It's best used before you curl your hair or to add longevity to your style.

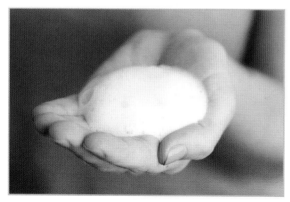

STYLING FOAM OR MOUSSE

This multitasking product can be used to add volume, not only to your roots, but also to the ends of your hair, while providing a light hold. It tames and helps shape your hair but doesn't leave it crunchy and dry. All hair types and textures can work with this type of product.

FIRM-HOLD GEL

This gel is designed to set your hair with maximum hold. You might see formal styles and up-dos make use of this product before blow-drying, to ensure the style lasts all night. If you have curly, rebellious hair, you could try using this gel for increased control.

THICKENING LOTION

This liquid, designed to coat each of your strands to make them fuller, is best for very fine hair that needs more body. It can double as a light-hold product as well.

VOLUMIZING POWDER

Sprinkle this fairy dust onto the roots of dry hair for added fullness. Some types of hair powder will reactivate throughout the day with a little heat and friction from your fingers. This provides a tousled, voluminous look.

CURL CREAM

This multipurpose product defines your curls while also providing a light hold – without weighing down your locks like other products may do. You can layer curl cream with a light- or firm-hold gel for maximum hold.

SEA-SALT SPRAY

Typically sprayed through the ends of your hair, sea-salt spray assists in creating a naturally wavy look. Those with naturally wavy or curly hair can achieve soft waves by using this mist. If you have straight hair, the spray will provide some texture and a touch of bend.

VOLUMIZING HAIRSPRAY

This hairspray is designed to promote volume. It usually has strong hold, to help amplify and maintain a voluminous style.

LIGHT-HOLD HAIRSPRAY

This hairspray is brushable and allows movement while also giving some hold. It should be heavy enough to retain a style, but without making your hair look or feel stiff.

Dry spray

Some recent lighter weight hairsprays are dry sprays. These provide hold without the stickiness that can sometimes accompany wet sprays.

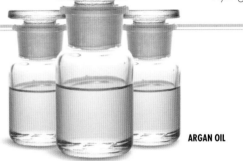

ARGAN OIL

MAXIMUM-HOLD HAIRSPRAY

This hairspray often includes an antihumidity ingredient that protects your hair from the environment to prolong your style. Some can feel stiff when in your hair; however, newer strong-hold sprays contain lighter ingredients that won't weigh down your hair. Max-hold sprays are typically used in formal styles or any style you don't want to move… at all.

ANTIFRIZZ SERUM

A product that combats frizz by surrounding your hair strands with a protective, moisturizing coating. Depending on the type of serum, it can be used on wet or dry hair, and effectively tames unruly hair. In some cases, it can help reduce the time your hair takes to dry.

ANTIHUMIDITY SERUM OR SPRAY

A styling product that protects your hair from the environment. It blocks moisture, preventing frizz, and can help smooth your hair and tame flyaways.

ARGAN OIL

This oil, produced from the kernels of a tree grown in Morocco, contains vitamins and essential fatty acids beneficial to your hair. A key ingredient in many products, it's useful for damaged hair or hair in need of moisture. It's easily absorbed, and can be used on wet or dry locks.

MOISTURIZING SERUM

This product – be it argan oil, an antifrizz serum, or any kind of serum that contains moisturizing ingredients – is used to soften and relax hair.

SHINE SPRAY

Used mostly as a finishing product, this mist is designed to enhance shine and bring life to dull hair. If you don't wash your hair every day, applying this spray to the ends of your hair, after using dry shampoo, can refresh your style. You can also use this spray before you gently comb through your curls.

SMOOTHING SERUM

This product, which could also be considered a moisturizing serum, typically contains an antifrizz or antihumidity property to coax wavy, coarse, or curly hair smooth and straight. Many serums also contain ingredients to help prevent future damage.

HEAT PROTECTOR

If you frequently use heated styling tools, you should frequently use this product. Heat protector normally comes in the form of a spray or cream, and contains oils to hydrate your hair. In addition, it helps protect your hair from humidity and may contain beneficial proteins.

SPRAY WAX

A new style of delivery for an old favourite, spray wax has a light to medium hold that's meant to add a touch of texture and grit to hair. Fine to medium hair types will benefit most from this thickening effect.

DEFINING PASTE

This is a lightweight finishing product, which is used to softly mould your hair. Shorter hairstyles can really reap the benefits of this paste. Applying a small amount throughout your hair adds texture.

TEXTURE PUTTY

Similar to defining paste, putty gives you a strong yet workable hold to your style. Texture putty works best for shaping shorter hair.

POMADE

This light-hold finishing product defines your strands and gives additional polish and shine.

Putty shades

Many types of putty are transparent and can be used on all hair types. But if the putty is light in colour, it's best to use it only on lighter coloured hair.

Styling Tools

You don't need a lot of specialized tools or equipment to style your hair, but a few basics will come in handy for lots of looks. Here are the commonly used hairstyling tools you might want to consider:

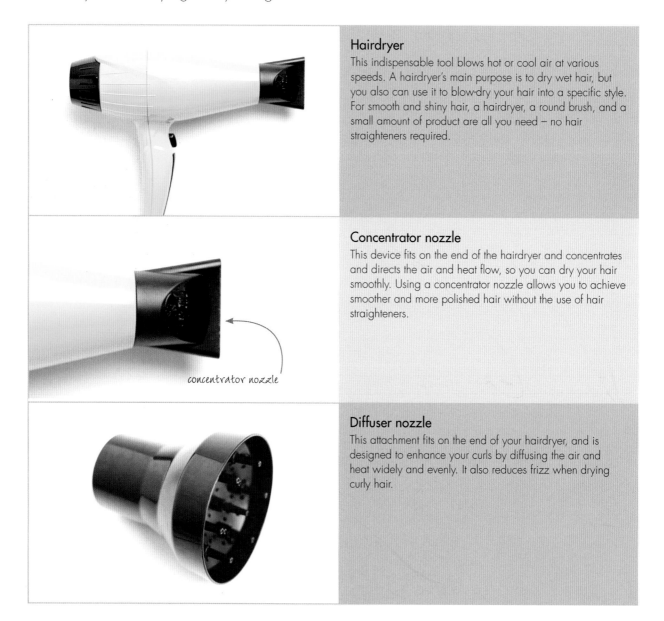

Hairdryer

This indispensable tool blows hot or cool air at various speeds. A hairdryer's main purpose is to dry wet hair, but you also can use it to blow-dry your hair into a specific style. For smooth and shiny hair, a hairdryer, a round brush, and a small amount of product are all you need – no hair straighteners required.

Concentrator nozzle

This device fits on the end of the hairdryer and concentrates and directs the air and heat flow, so you can dry your hair smoothly. Using a concentrator nozzle allows you to achieve smoother and more polished hair without the use of hair straighteners.

concentrator nozzle

Diffuser nozzle

This attachment fits on the end of your hairdryer, and is designed to enhance your curls by diffusing the air and heat widely and evenly. It also reduces frizz when drying curly hair.

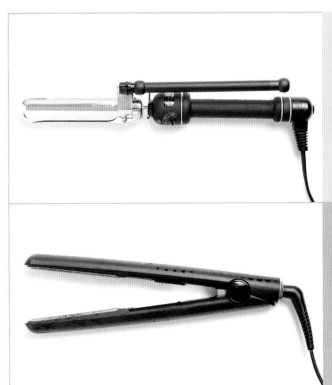

Curling tongs

This handheld tool has a barrel at one end that heats up. You coil your hair around the hot barrel, close the clamp to keep your hair against the barrel, hold for a few seconds, and unclamp for curly locks. Multiple barrel sizes are available, ranging from 1cm to 5cm in diameter. The larger the barrel, the larger the curls.

Hair straighteners

Also called straightening irons, this tool also uses intense heat to style your hair. It has two ceramic plates that close together, sandwiching your hair in between, to smooth and flatten your hair. Straighteners can get extremely hot, often reaching temperatures upwards of 200°C.

Other heated helpers you might find include curling wands, three-barrel curling tongs, and crimpers.

A curling wand is basically curling tongs without a clamp. It is great for getting mermaid waves.

Three-barrel curling tongs typically have two barrels on the bottom and one on the top. Pressing your hair between the barrels creates soft, uniform waves.

Crimpers kink your hair into sharp, zigzag waves. First popular in the 1980s, this look has made a comeback on runways and at parties.

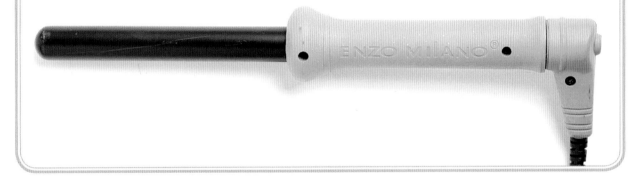

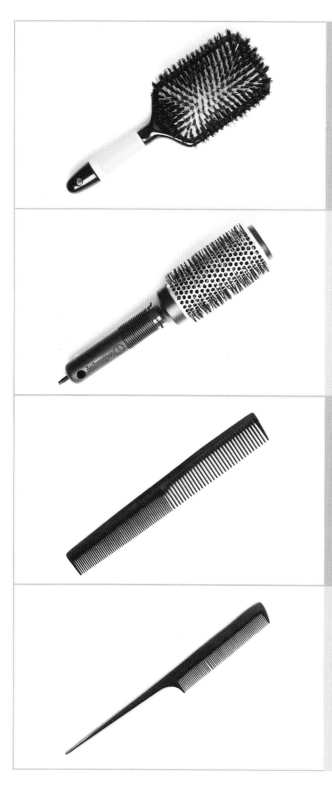

Paddle brush
This large, flat brush is used to detangle and help reduce drying time when blow-drying. The bristles are designed to be gentle on wet and dry hair alike. It can even give you a bit of a scalp massage when you brush thoroughly.

Round brush
This brush will soon become your favourite. It's essential for smoothing, taming, and curling your hair while blow-drying. Opt for a vented version if you can find one. There are many sizes of round brush, yielding different styles. A smaller brush produces a curlier look at the middle and ends of your hair, while a larger size is used mainly to smooth the hair, adding a slight bend at the ends.

Comb
This general comb has many uses. It's best to have one that's heat resistant, so you can use it to guide and keep your hair smooth while you use heated styling tools. A good general comb can also be used to mould hair into up-dos.

Tail comb
This comb has small teeth at one end and a straight, pointy pick at the other end. The pointy end is helpful for precisely parting and sectioning your hair before styling.

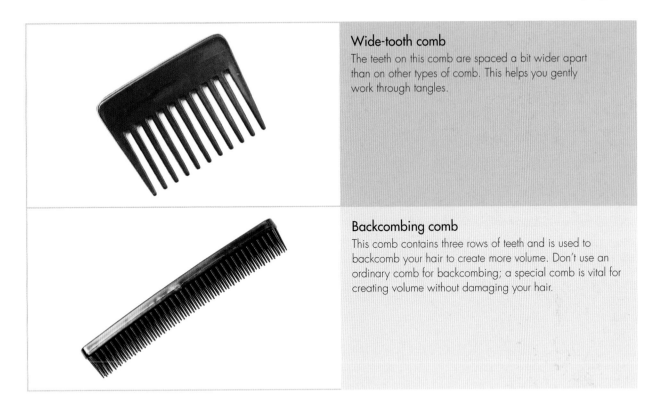

Wide-tooth comb
The teeth on this comb are spaced a bit wider apart than on other types of comb. This helps you gently work through tangles.

Backcombing comb
This comb contains three rows of teeth and is used to backcomb your hair to create more volume. Don't use an ordinary comb for backcombing; a special comb is vital for creating volume without damaging your hair.

Backcombing brushes and vent brushes are two other types of brushes to try.

Backcombing brushes usually contain a mix of nylon and boar bristles and are used, just like combs, to add volume and texture.

Vent brushes have slots in the body of the brush, between the bristles. When you use a vent brush as you blow-dry your hair, air flows through these vents and around your hair, enabling you to dry it faster.

Styling Aids

Used alongside the basic styling tools and products, these styling aids are often crucial for creating – and maintaining – your look:

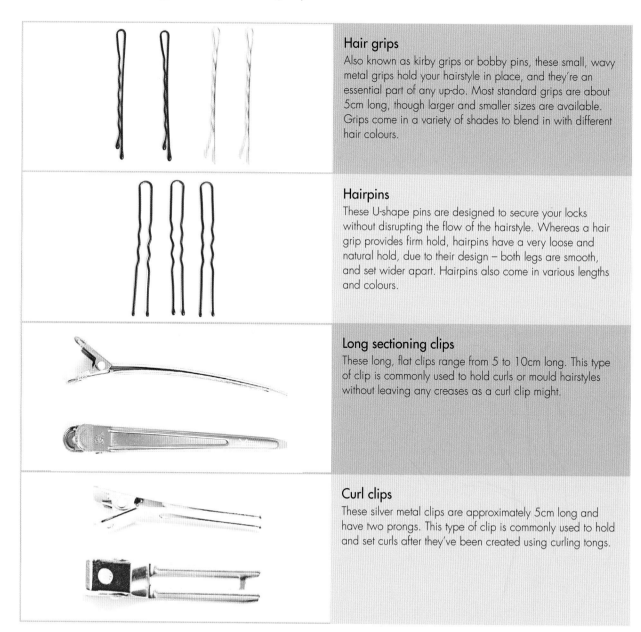

Hair grips

Also known as kirby grips or bobby pins, these small, wavy metal grips hold your hairstyle in place, and they're an essential part of any up-do. Most standard grips are about 5cm long, though larger and smaller sizes are available. Grips come in a variety of shades to blend in with different hair colours.

Hairpins

These U-shape pins are designed to secure your locks without disrupting the flow of the hairstyle. Whereas a hair grip provides firm hold, hairpins have a very loose and natural hold, due to their design – both legs are smooth, and set wider apart. Hairpins also come in various lengths and colours.

Long sectioning clips

These long, flat clips range from 5 to 10cm long. This type of clip is commonly used to hold curls or mould hairstyles without leaving any creases as a curl clip might.

Curl clips

These silver metal clips are approximately 5cm long and have two prongs. This type of clip is commonly used to hold and set curls after they've been created using curling tongs.

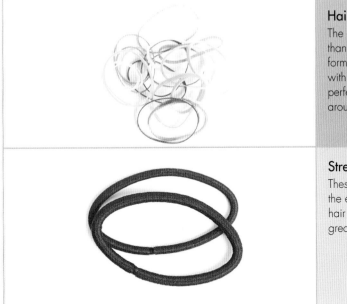

Hair elastics

The clear version of these stretchy bands, often no larger than 1–2cm in diameter, are commonly used in up-styles and formal hairdos. Because they're clear, they camouflage well with your hair. Coloured elastics are also available and are perfect for adding a pop of colour to the end of a plait or around ponytails.

Stretchy ponytail bands

These larger, stretchy bands contain a fabric coating over the elastic. They come in different sizes to suit a variety of hair thicknesses and in a wide variety of colours. They're great for securing ponytails for maximum hold.

Two other styling aids you might find helpful when creating hairstyles at home are fabric hairbands and bun sponges.

Fabric hairbands are a modern, decorative version of a hair tie. They come in countless designs, providing a quick and easy splash of colour in your hair.

Bun sponges help you form the perfect bun. Pull your ponytail through the centre hole of this doughnut-shaped sponge and then pin your hair around the doughnut to create a full, round bun. If you have trouble forming a voluminous bun with your hair, try one of these. They're available in different colours and sizes.

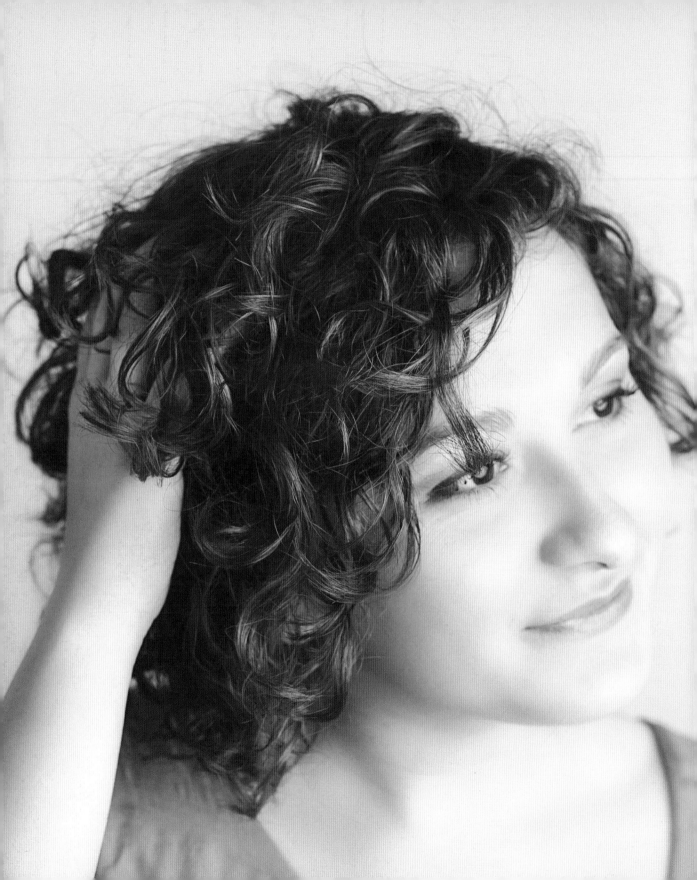

Hairstyling
Basics

Just like you can't build a house without any bricklaying or carpentry skills, you shouldn't expect to create perfect hairdos without first learning the basics of hairstyling. This section gives you the building blocks necessary for many of the styles in this book, including how to add volume, tame frizz, and achieve shiny locks.

It's easy to overlook the importance of prepping your hair before beginning a style. But how you prep your hair determines how it behaves in the finished style. If you don't pay attention to this stage, you won't be able to achieve your desired style. Your hair type also determines what kind of prep you need. If you have curly hair, for example, you'll want to use heavy, moisturizing products before styling, while someone with straight, fine hair will need a cocktail of volume builders to boost their style. Whatever your hair type, texture, or length, here you'll find the best way to get your tresses into shape.

Adding Volume

If your locks are more limp and lifeless than you'd like them to be, you can boost them with additional volume. How you build body and create fullness will depend on the type of hair you have.

FINE HAIR

If you have fine hair, whether it's straight or wavy, yours requires the most manipulation to create volume. First, thoroughly towel dry your hair. Apply a thickening serum, and comb it through your hair from the roots to the tips. Next, add a root lifter (either a foam or a spray type will work) to your scalp in the crown area. Lastly, apply a styling foam or a mousse from the middle to the ends of your hair, for voluminous hold in your finished style.

MEDIUM HAIR

If your hair isn't particularly fine or thick, you'll still have a bit of work to do to add volume. For straight hair, follow the directions for adding volume to fine hair, but skip the thickening serum, as your hair is thick enough not to need it.

If your hair is wavy, you'll need to use different products. When your hair is still damp, add a root lifter to your scalp in the crown area. You also can add a light moisturizing serum for moisture and control of your waves. The serum helps alleviate frizz when you're adding volume. Then finish with an application of mousse to the middle and ends of your hair.

THICK HAIR

Thick hair requires the most moisture. With straight hair, you might be able to skip a heavy, moisturizing serum and opt for a lighter one. However, the volumizing process is the same.

While your hair is damp, apply a moisturizing serum. This will penetrate the hair shaft and retain moisture. Next, you'll seal in the moisture, while also creating volume. Use a mixture of sculpting gel and shine spray to help with moisture retention and hold. Lastly, you can add some mousse or a bit more gel to the ends of your hair, for maximum volume.

Stick to the roots

With thick hair, extra volume usually isn't needed from the middle to the ends of your hair. So you can skip the final mousse or extra gel stage if you feel you have enough thickness already.

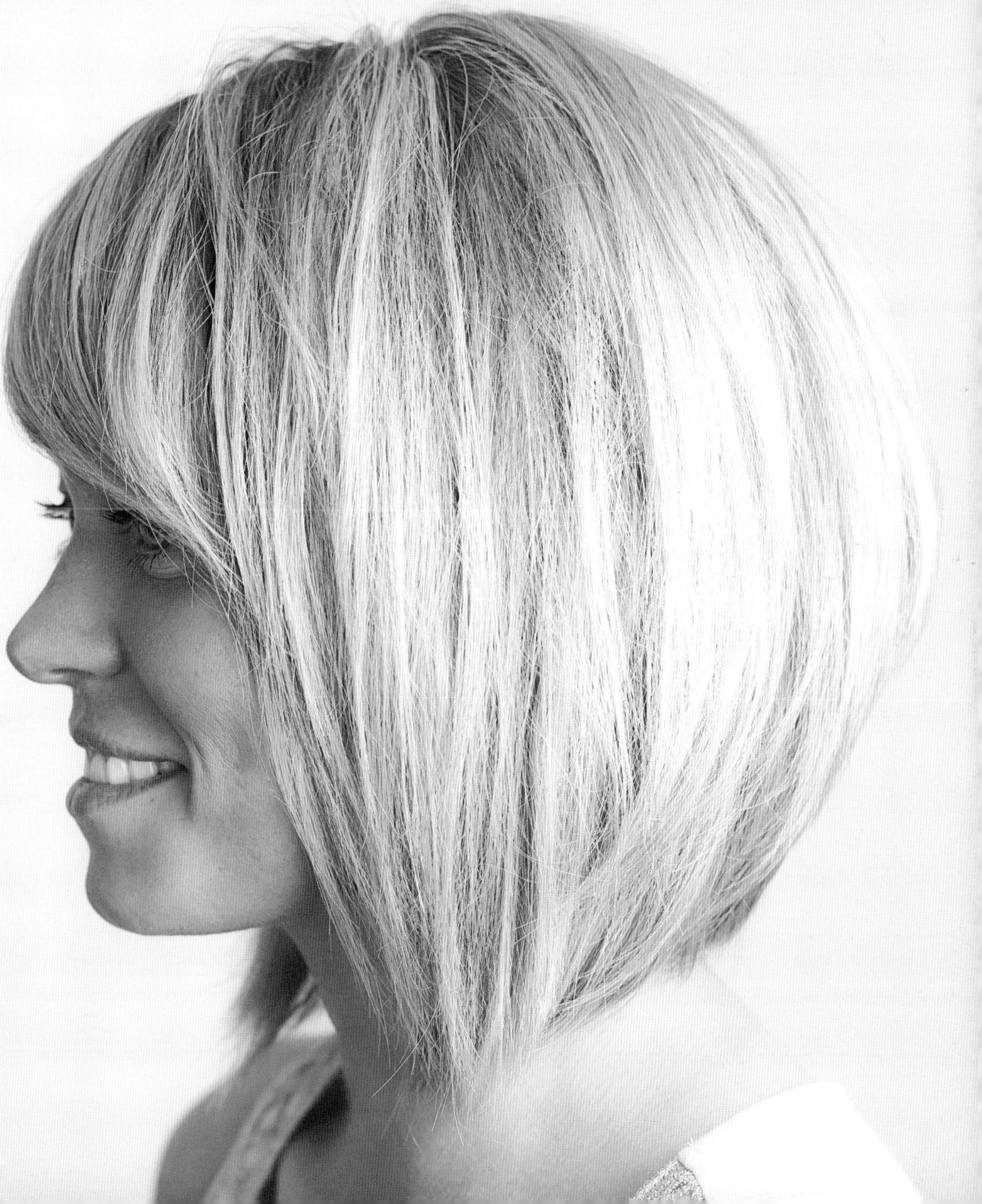

Taming Frizz

Frizz can ruin an otherwise lovely look, and to make matters worse, it can be one of the hardest hairstyle problems to fix. Taming frizz has to do primarily with the condition your hair is in. The most important consideration is the moisture level of your hair.

FINE HAIR

If you have fine hair and frizz, it's most likely due to breakage around your hairline or new, baby hairs growing in that area.

To tame frizz in fine hair, you can first use a light moisturizing serum to address any lack of moisture. Then you can apply a moisture sealant such as Argan oil to the middle and ends of your hair, to lock in moisture.

If absolutely necessary, you could add an antifrizz serum after applying the moisture sealant, but before you blow-dry your hair. If your hair still looks as if it has flyaways, use a bit of defining paste to press down the flyaways after your hair is dry.

MEDIUM AND THICK HAIR

Medium, wavy hair and thick, curly hair need the most moisture, and are typically the most prone to frizz. If you have either of these types of hair, first use a moisturizing serum when your hair is damp; apply it from the middle down to the ends of your hair. Next, use an antifrizz serum on the middle and ends of your hair to tame the frizz and act as an antihumidity barrier.

Blow-dry your hair, using a paddle brush to pull your hair smooth while drying. Be sure to dry from the roots to the ends, pushing your hair cuticle downwards to avoid creating additional frizz.

If you prefer to dry your hair upside down, make sure you are still directing the hairdryer along your hair from the roots to the ends. Blow-drying hair in the wrong direction is one of the most common mistakes that leads to frizz.

Keep it light

When working with fine hair, be careful not to overload it with heavy silicone and waxes. Layering products – and choosing the right products – gives the best results. If possible, use only high-quality styling products.

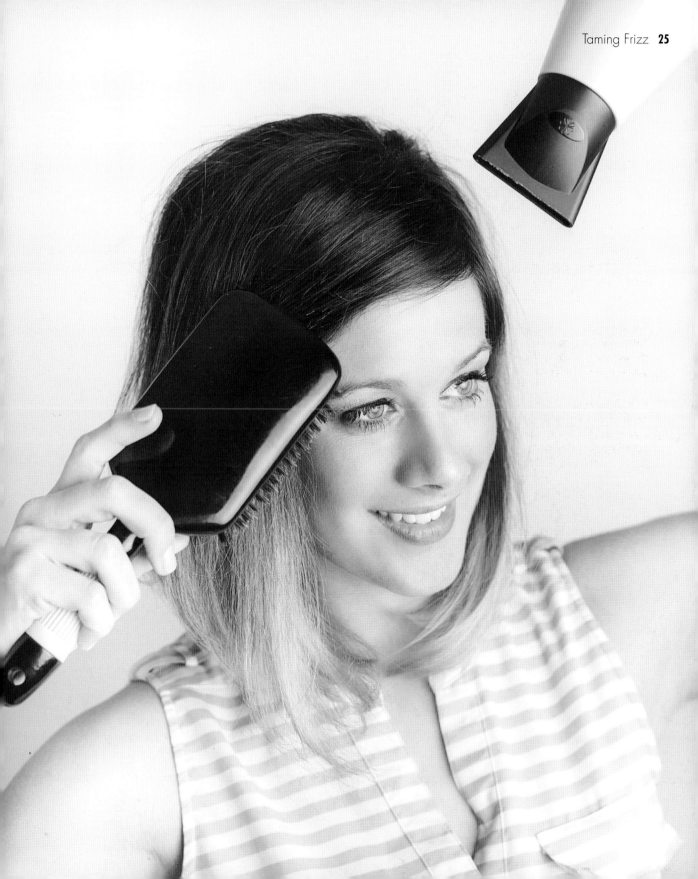

Getting Shiny Hair

One reason hair isn't shiny could be that it's unhealthy due to lack of moisture, or it has suffered some sort of damage. Hot styling tools and the chemicals used in hair colours and other products can strip your hair of its natural oils. For the same reason, washing your hair every day isn't necessarily a good thing. Frequent washing removes oils that are necessary to keep your hair in its optimal condition. With the combination of repeated washing and the use of heated tools and various chemical treatments, it's no wonder your hair can look dull.

TIPS FOR HEALTHY SHINE

The first step back to silky, shiny strands is to evaluate your shampoo and conditioner. Try using a moisturizing or repairing shampoo and conditioning system to help your hair get back to its natural healthy state. Using a moisturizing serum and/or heat protector on your hair when it's damp, before you blow-dry, can prevent any further moisture loss.

You might want to forgo your hairdryer if your hair is in a fragile condition. If you're trying to restore your hair's health but need to use a heated styling tool, it's best to skip the hairdryer and just use the heated tool on naturally dried hair. If you blow-dry your hair when it's damaged, and then use tongs or straighteners directly afterwards, you increase the risk of further damage.

Although maintaining your hair's optimal health is the best way to encourage shine, you can help it along by adding a shine mist or serum to the ends of your hair, after your style is complete. With either product, use it in moderation and only from the middle to the ends of your hair.

Ingredient nasties

Look at the ingredient lists to check what's in the products you use on your hair and that they don't contain fillers. You want pure ingredients for optimal hair health. Heavy silicones or waxes can zap the shine right out of your hair.

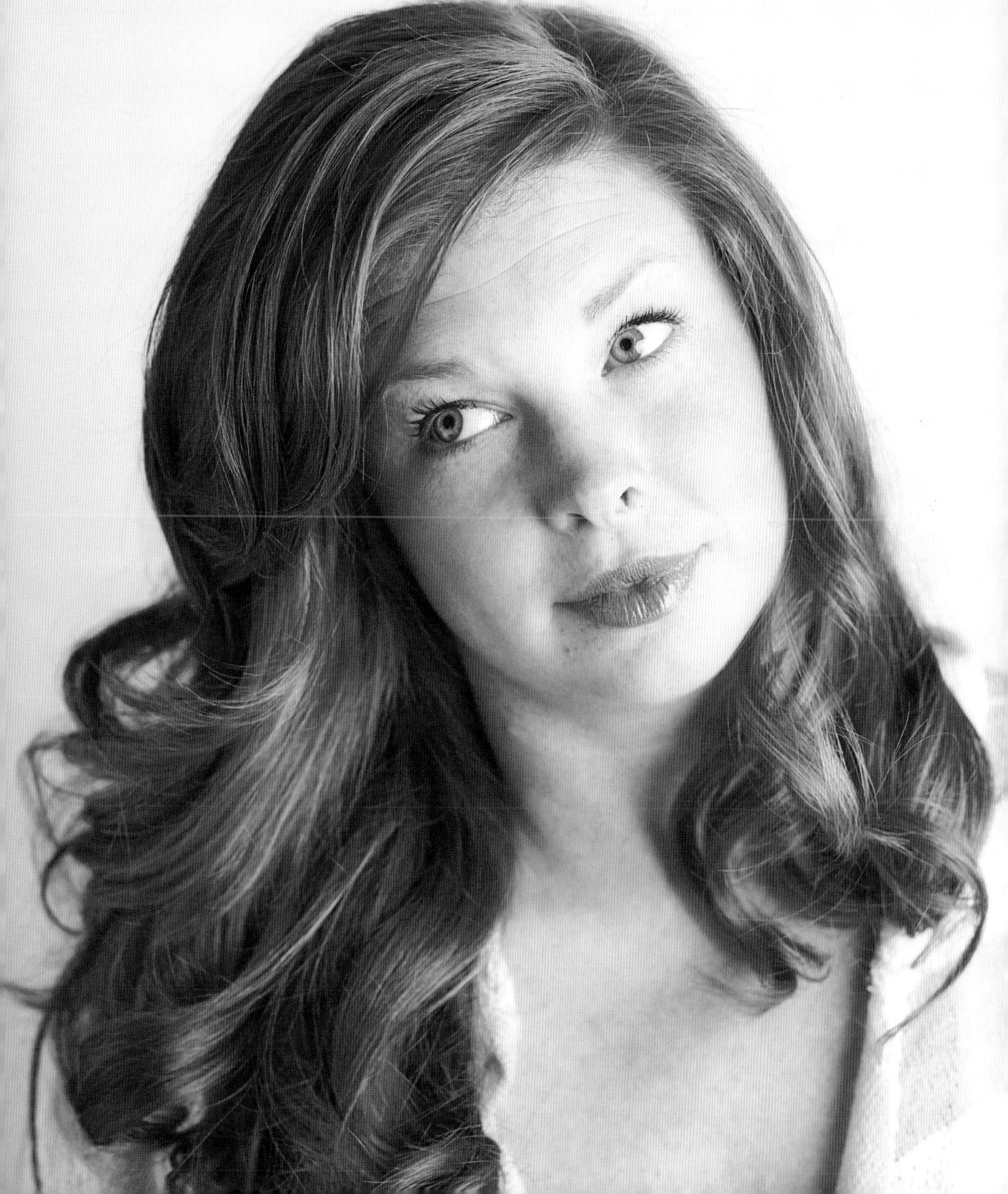

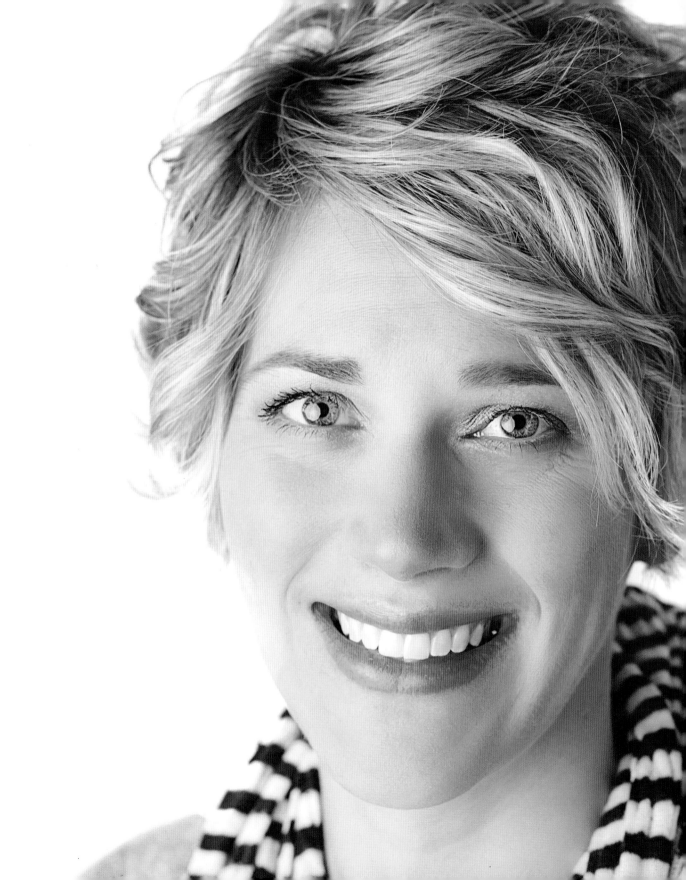

Styles for Short Hair

If you want quick and easy to manage hair, a short style can be the answer. However, it's all too common for someone to cut their hair short, and then to stick with the same look day after day.

It can be exciting to get your hair chopped into a new, stylish crop – but that's just the beginning. Take the time to learn how to style it and your short haircut can reach its full, versatile potential. In the following pages, you'll find different ways to style your short cut that bring out the best in your hair.

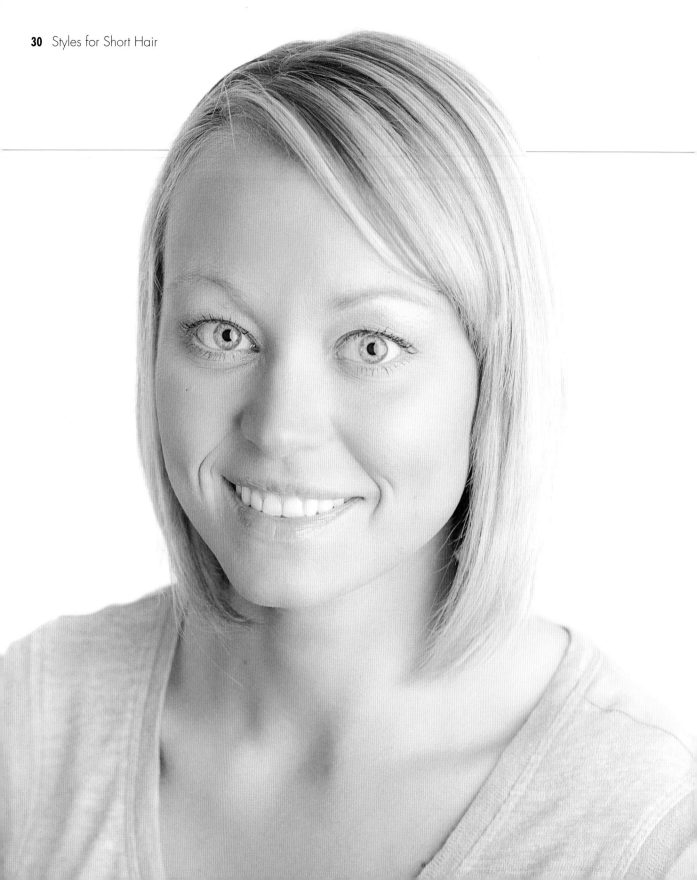

Sleek and Straight

SHORT

This style should be a staple in your hairstyle arsenal. All types of hair can achieve the sleek look with the right products, tools, and skills. For straight hair, use straighteners for smoothing flyaway hairs. If you have waves or curls, you'll need to tame these to get the silky look. You can wear this look anywhere – from a business meeting to a night out clubbing.

Thoroughly towel dry your hair and then add product. For straight or fine hair, use both root lifter and volumizing mousse for extra movement. With medium to thicker strands with more texture, condition hair with moisturizing oil, then add a serum to avoid frizz. Wavy- and curly-haired types can also add a volumizing spray at the roots to boost volume on top.

TOOLS NEEDED

- hairdryer
- concentrator nozzle
- sectioning clips
- hair straighteners
- antihumidity serum (optional)
- heat-resistant comb
- heat protection spray
- light- to medium-hold hairspray
- paddle brush

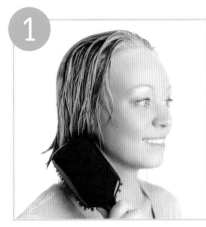

1 Start with thoroughly towel-dried hair. Apply product as necessary, depending on your hair type, and gently brush through your hair with a paddle brush.

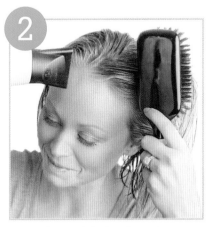

2 Using the paddle brush and your hairdryer fitted with a concentrator nozzle, blow-dry your hair from the roots to the ends in opposite directions, creating soft volume, until your hair is dry.

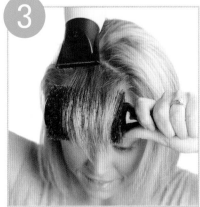

3 If you have a fringe, blow-dry that area until any kinks are relaxed. It's best to tame these while your hair is wet. When it's dry, hair is more difficult to mould.

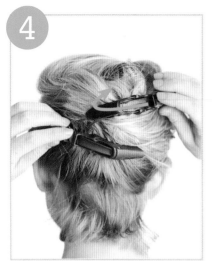

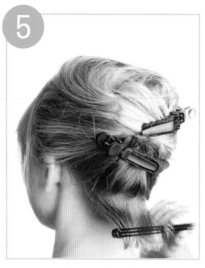

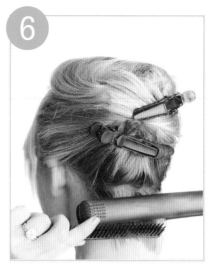

When your hair is completely dry, separate out a section of hair at the nape of your neck, about 2.5cm up from your hairline. Pull the rest up and out of the way and secure it with clips.

Spray your hair with a heat protection spray to prevent damage. Separate a subsection of the loose hair about 5cm wide. Place a heat-resistant comb beneath this section, lifting it about 45 degrees from where it falls.

Close the straighteners on your hair as close to the base of your scalp as you can, and slowly glide them down, tilting under slightly at the end. Repeat on another 5cm section and continue around the whole of the nape of your neck.

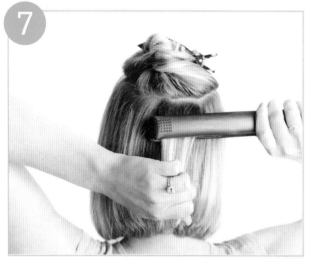

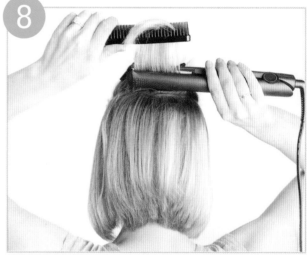

Separate another horizontal section about 2.5cm wide above the one you just straightened, and repeat steps 5 and 6. Continue with this method until you reach the crown of your head.

At the crown, hold your hair at a 90-degree angle when straightening to add volume: insert the comb at 90 degrees under the hair at your crown, place the straighteners close to the scalp, and glide slowly to the ends in a fluid motion. Each motion takes 4 to 6 seconds, depending on hair length.

9

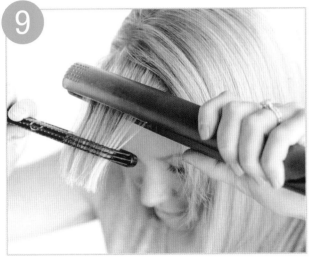

If you have a fringe, you can now straighten it. Insert the comb beneath your fringe at a 45-degree angle – just enough to lift the hair off your forehead – and smooth with the straighteners.

10

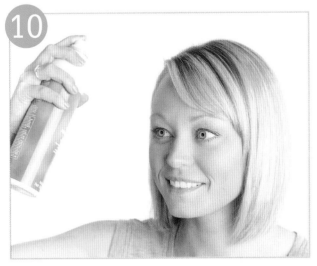

Now finish with a light- to medium-hold hairspray. If you have wavy or curly hair, you might want to add some additional humidity resistance with antihumidity serum.

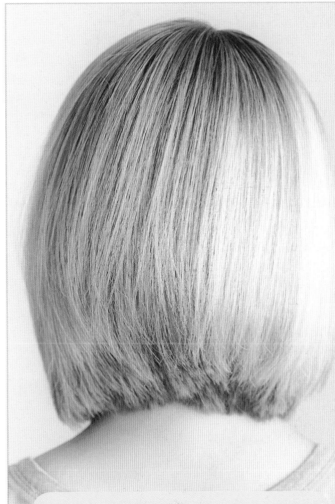

Getting the best results

It's a common misconception that you need to glide the straighteners down your hair very quickly multiple times to achieve smooth, shiny tresses. To use this technique correctly, it's best to move slowly and steadily down your hair just the once. If needed, you can run the straighteners over a second time for stubborn, coarse hair.

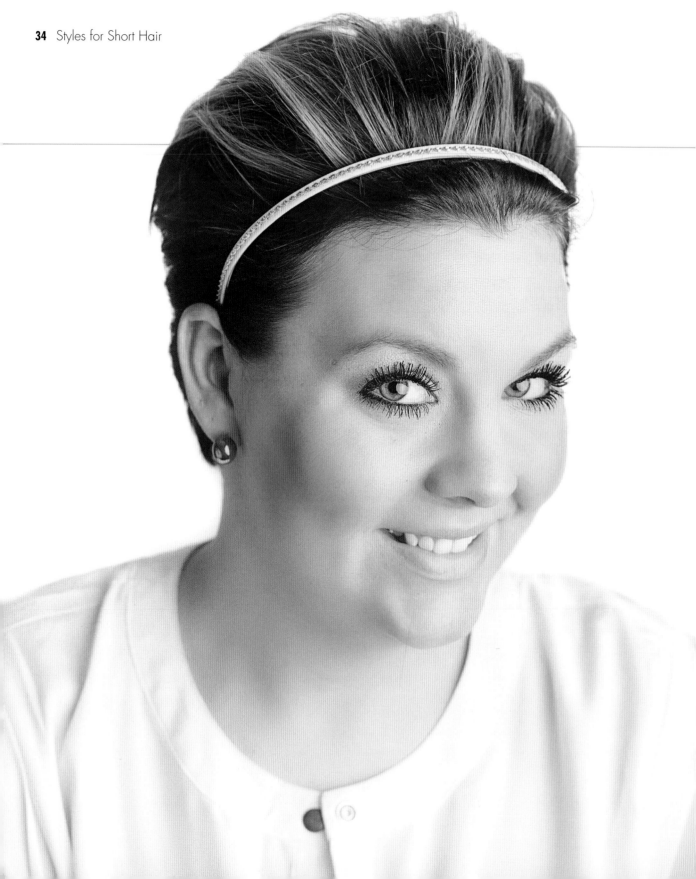

Short Hair Blow-Dry

This style is a polished, easy, everyday look that lasts. Wash and blow-dry your hair on Monday, and then add simple adjustments to transform your style into multiple hairdos. This blow-dry is one of the most versatile hairstyles, easily taking you from the school run to a dinner date.

All hair types work with this style. Hair should be thoroughly towel dried before applying products. Fine-hair types should use a cocktail of root lifter and volumizing mousse for extra bounce. If you have medium to thick hair, add volume and hold with a light-hold gel or styling glaze, and avoid frizz with a smoothing serum. Those with thick, coarse, or curly tresses should first soften with a moisturizing serum, then add mousse or gel for hold and shine.

TOOLS NEEDED

- hairdryer
- concentrator nozzle
- sectioning clips
- defining paste
- medium-hold hairspray
- paddle brush
- round brush
- wide-tooth comb

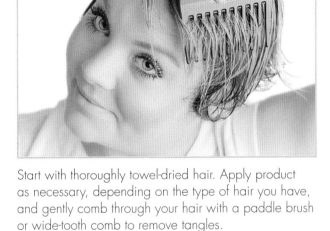

Start with thoroughly towel-dried hair. Apply product as necessary, depending on the type of hair you have, and gently comb through your hair with a paddle brush or wide-tooth comb to remove tangles.

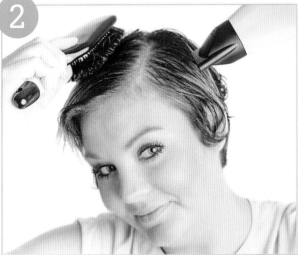

Fit the concentrator nozzle to your hairdryer for the correct heat flow. Then use the paddle brush and hairdryer to dry your hair from the roots to the ends in opposite directions to create volume.

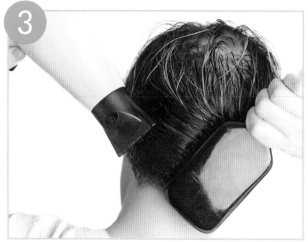

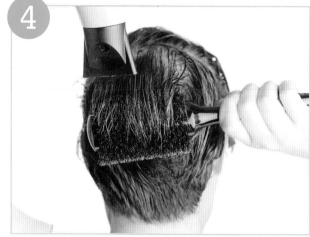

As you're moving to the back of your head and pushing your paddle brush back and forth, blow all your hair to one side and let it naturally shape around your head. After you've removed most of the moisture from that side, switch to the other side, and continue pushing your hair to the opposite side to let it naturally gain a little bend. Continue drying your hair until it's about 80 per cent dry.

Clip up all except a horizontal section of hair at the nape of the neck, about 5cm wide (or high enough to get enough hair to wrap around the brush). Insert the round brush at a 45-degree angle under the subsection, and using the concentrator nozzle, medium heat, and firm tension, gently glide to the ends. At the ends, rotate the brush a couple of times with the heat still on it to enhance the curl. Repeat with the sections of hair above this section until you reach the crown.

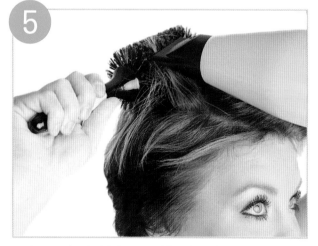

At the crown, hold the round brush under your hair at a 90-degree angle from your scalp to create maximum volume. Use the brush and hairdryer as you did for the rest of your hair to create polished volume at the crown.

The perfect fringe

If you have a full fringe, use the round brush in a forwards motion, let it cool for a few seconds on the brush, and then release your hair. This should ensure your fringe lies neatly. If you have a side-swept fringe, it's best to round brush forwards first with firm tension, and then slightly tilt your brush to the side, with the concentrator firmly pressed against the brush. You can blow-dry your hair all the way to the ends and drop, without letting it cool.

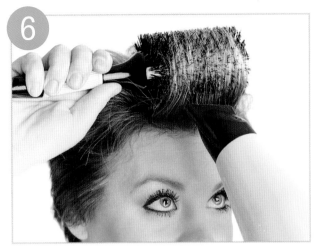

Along your front hairline, direct your hair at 90 degrees up and back, away from the face. Backcomb your hair at the hairline to add volume around your face if you have fine hair.

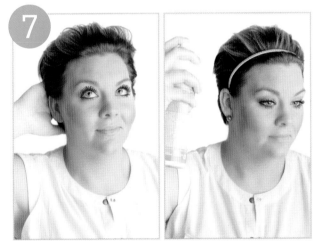

Use defining paste to smooth the sides and finish with a medium-hold hairspray. For a little extra sparkle, add a headband to dress up this style.

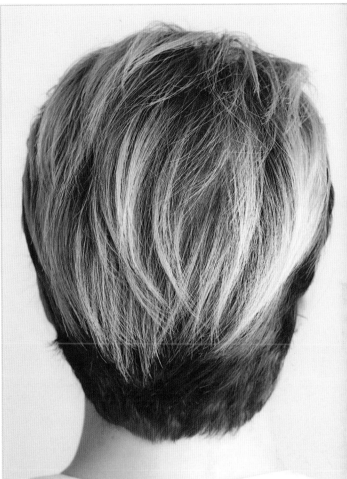

A sleek look

If you have tapered or shorter hair at the back of the head, try this technique to help hair look just as polished at the back as at the front. When your hair is 80 per cent dry, clip the longer hair up. Start above the bone just above the nape of the neck. Push the brush against the head, place the concentrator nozzle on the brush, and roll hair from the roots to the ends.

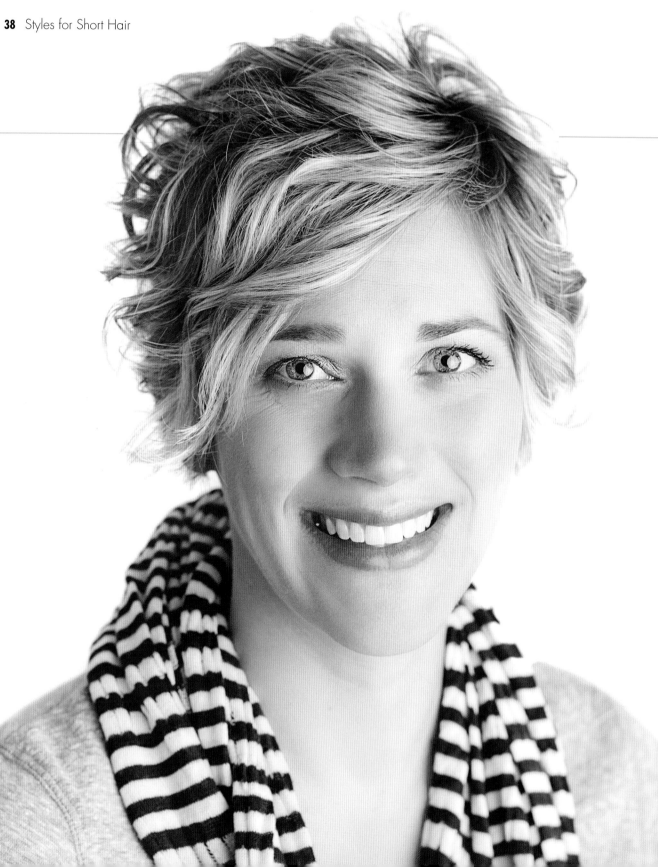

Tousled Texture

SHORT

Anyone with naturally curly or wavy locks will love this style, which tames yet enhances your hair's texture. It's amazing what the right type and amount of product can do for your style – you can go from drab to fab in about 10 minutes. Although this is a simple hairdo to create, it's very versatile, and easy to dress up for special occasions.

If you have fine and/or straight hair, you might not have enough natural texture to create this look. To begin this style, you want your hair to be slightly damp. You can towel dry it, but it should still have some moisture in it when you apply product.

TOOLS NEEDED

- antifrizz or moisturizing serum
- antihumidity hairspray
- hairdryer
- diffuser nozzle
- hair grips (optional)
- curl cream
- defining paste

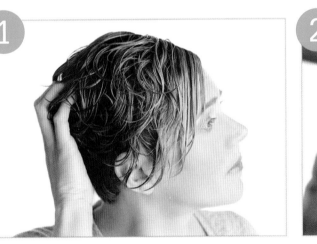

1 Start with damp hair. Squeeze a small amount of antifrizz or moisturizing serum into your palms and rub them together to distribute the serum. Apply to your hair from your ears downwards. To avoid an oily look, don't apply in the root area.

2 To enhance your natural texture, apply a dollop of curl cream about 2.5cm in diameter evenly through your hair, again avoiding the scalp.

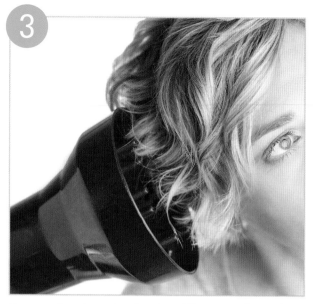

Use your hairdryer, fitted with a diffuser nozzle, on low heat to enhance your curl but minimize frizz. Continue until the hair is about 75 per cent dry if you have curly hair. If your hair is wavy, dry to about 90 per cent.

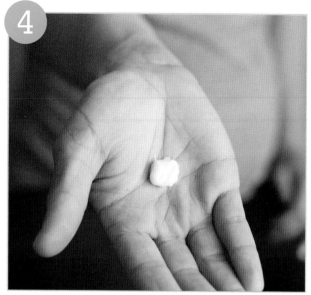

When your hair is dried to the desired stage, it's time to apply some defining paste. Squeeze a dollop about 2cm in diameter into the palm of your hand.

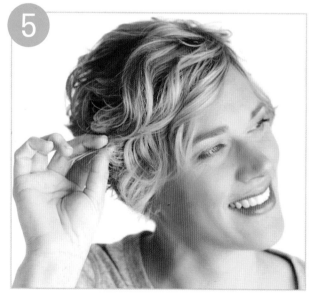

Now get creative: pick and choose individual sections of hair that are frizzy or unruly, and glide down them with your fingers coated in the paste.

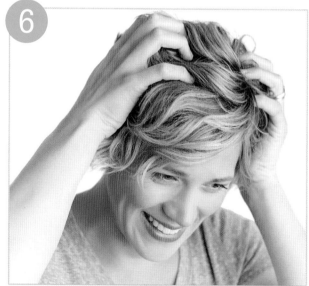

After you've applied paste to individual sections, you can add another dollop of paste and scrunch it into your hair for additional bounce.

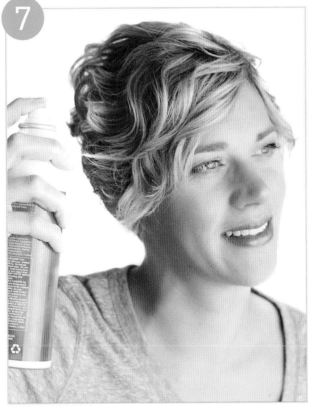

To finish, spray your hair with an antihumidity hairspray to keep your style intact and frizz-free.

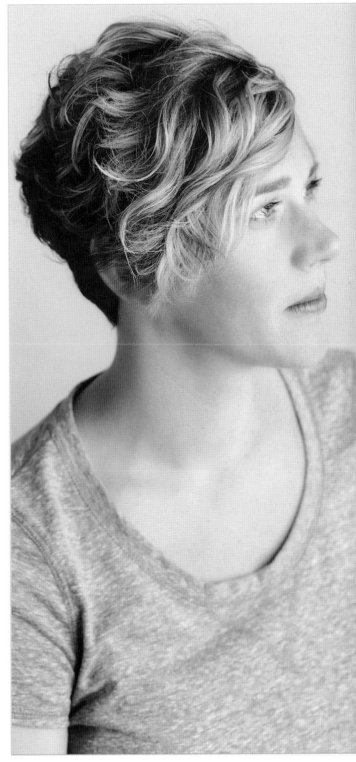

Tidying up

Curly hair tends to shrink when it's dry, so the fringe area commonly hangs down over the eyes when it's blow-dried. To avoid this, you can pin your fringe away from your face with hair grips, going with the natural flow of your wave or curl, and gently pinning the fringe back on one side.

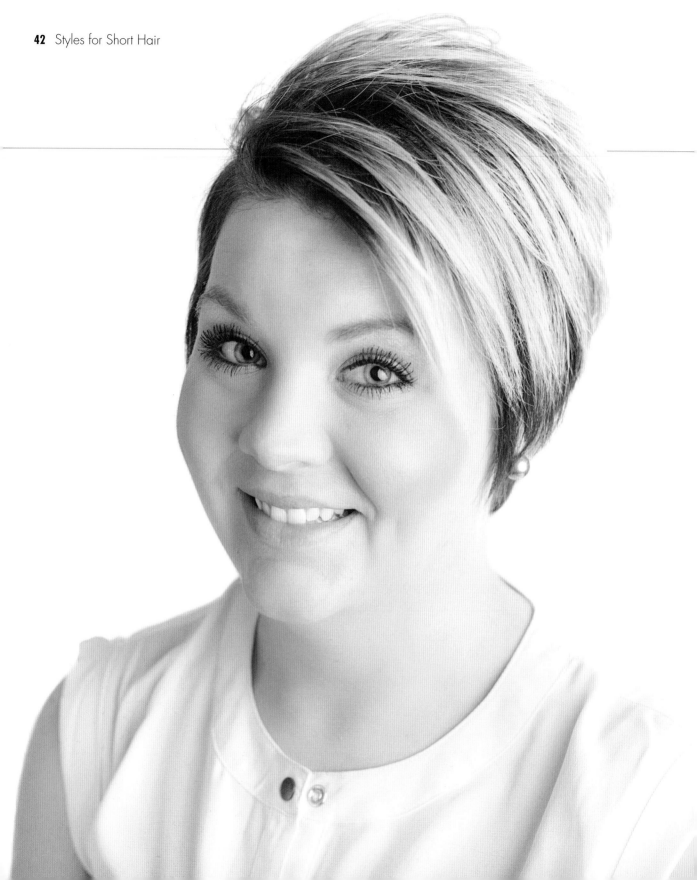

Sleek Look

SHORT

Short hair is often styled the same way day after day. Because of its length, there aren't as many ways to style shorter locks as there are for longer hair. But if you want to add some variety to your repertoire, this is the style for you. This sleek hairdo looks great anywhere, from a chic lunch date to the red carpet. You can wear it either styled wet or blow-dried. The most flattering version is blow-dried, which provides some extra volume.

TOOLS NEEDED

- hairdryer
- concentrator nozzle
- sectioning clips
- firm-hold styling gel
- medium- to firm-hold hairspray
- root lifter
- round brush (you might need a variety of sizes for different results)
- water spray bottle
- wide-tooth comb

All hair types can sport this look. However, it's best suited to fine or medium hair types that are straight or wavy. Wash your hair with moisturizing shampoo and conditioner to help reduce frizz. If you have fine hair, be sure to thoroughly rinse the conditioner from your scalp. When drying, use a towel to remove the excess moisture, and gently squeeze your hair, don't rub it. (Rubbing strands together can contribute to breakage.)

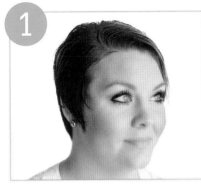

Start with towel-dried hair. Apply root lifter to the hair in the crown area, spraying it directly towards your scalp.

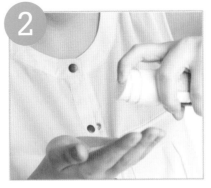

Next, apply a dollop of firm-hold styling gel about 2cm to 2.5cm in diameter to the middle and ends of your hair.

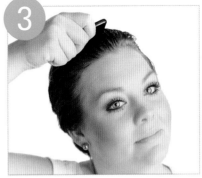

Use a wide-tooth comb to evenly distribute the product through the hair, while gently detangling.

▶

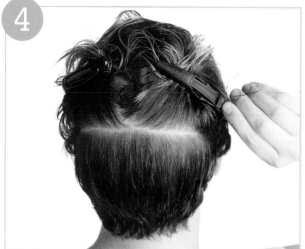

Your hair should still be damp at this point. If it's not, lightly spray it with a water spray bottle. Clip up all your hair except for a small horizontal 5cm section at the nape of your neck. If your hair is tapered at the neck, clip up all but the lowest 5cm layer you can clip.

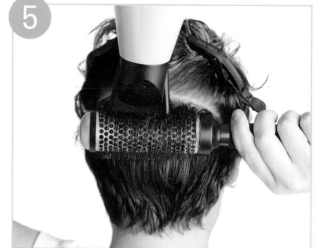

Insert a round brush beneath the bottom layer of the 5cm section and hold your hairdryer, with the concentrator nozzle attached, against the brush. Blow-dry downwards while rolling the ends for maximum body. Repeat, working around your head along the bottom layer, until your hair is dry. Unclip a second horizontal section and repeat.

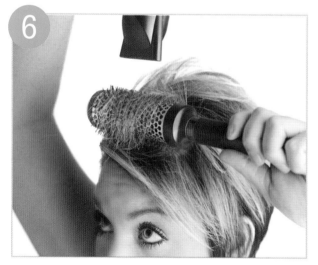

When you've reached the top section, insert the round brush and lift the hair at a 90-degree angle for maximum volume as you blow-dry.

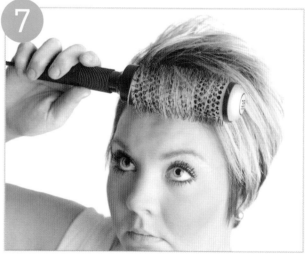

At your front hairline, working in a section 5cm wide, spray your hair with water if necessary to make it very damp. Hold the front section of hair outwards at 90 degrees from your scalp. Insert the round brush beneath your hair and blow it towards your face.

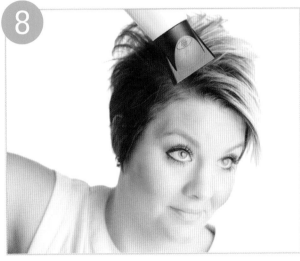

Repeat step 7 along the rest of your hairline at the sides, continuing to blow your hair towards your face while parting it on one side and pushing it slightly forwards.

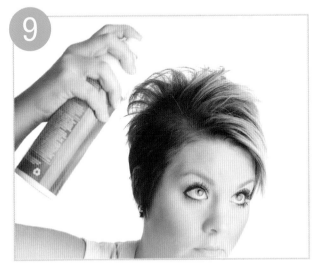

To finish, spray your hair with either a medium- or firm-hold hairspray. It's best to use an antihumidity spray with maximum hold, so your style won't deflate.

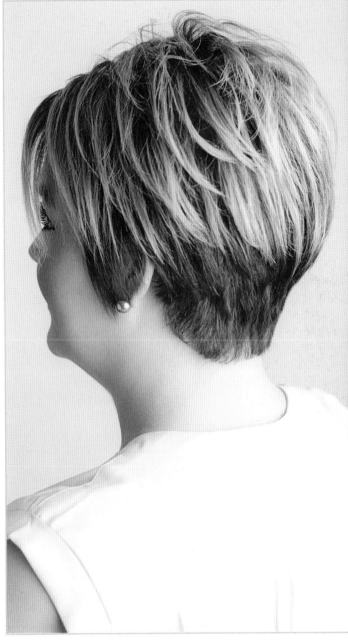

Extra body

Try backcombing at the front of your hair and in the crown area for extra volume.

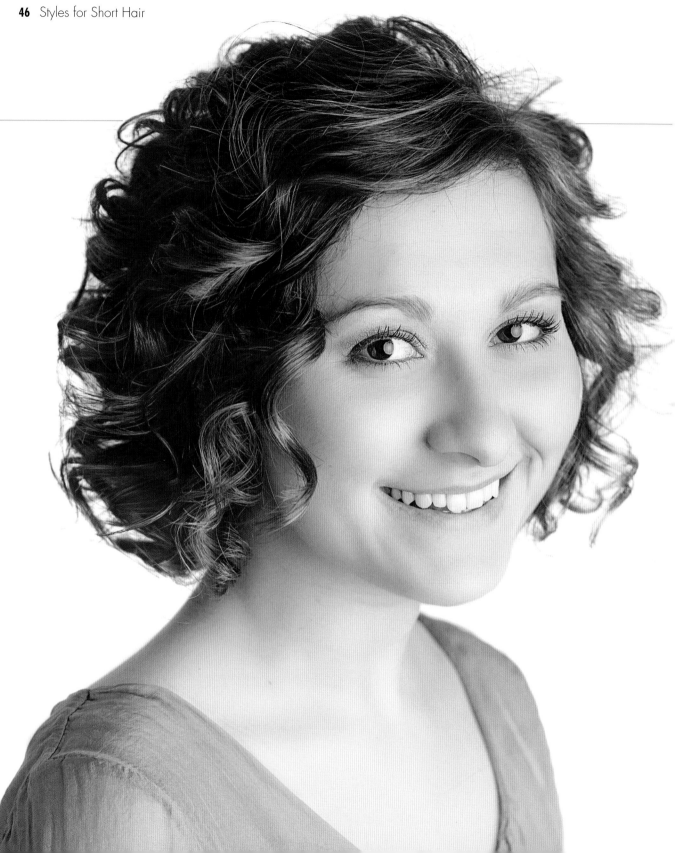

Curly Girl

SHORT

This style shows the versatility of short hair, combining the bounce and sassiness of a short cut with a bit of sophisticated polish. You could wear these soft coils while out running errands, or spiced up with a little volume for a dinner date. The style works with all types of hair, though naturally textured hair won't require as much prep time.

If you have straight hair, use volumizing mousse to plump up those strands and give your tongs something to grasp on to. Wavy and curly textures can use a moisturizing serum on damp hair and a light-hold product afterwards, such as a sculpting or setting lotion, or volumizing mousse.

TOOLS NEEDED

- hairdryer
- concentrator (nozzle)
- sectioning clips
- comb
- curling cream
- curling tongs
- defining paste
- paddle brush
- round brush (optional)
- shine spray

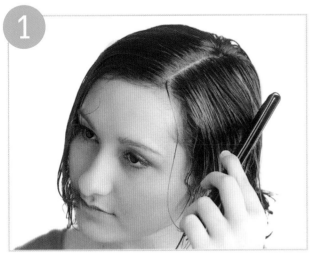

Start with towel-dried hair that's slightly damp. Apply product as necessary, depending on your hair type, and gently distribute through your hair with a comb or paddle brush. Prepping your hair before you blow-dry is vital to the finished style.

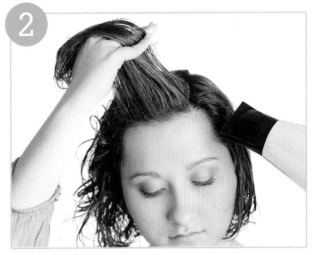

Using the concentrator nozzle on your hairdryer, dry your hair in opposite directions for volume. Remember to also continue drying your hair from the roots to the ends while you're flipping your hair back and forth. This helps smooth out knots and flyaway hairs.

▶

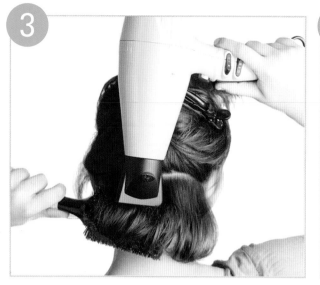

With short hair, it's unlikely that you'll need to curl the area at the nape of your neck. It's best to try to smooth this area while you're blow-drying. You could add some shape by inserting a round brush underneath your hair and rolling it down the back of your head.

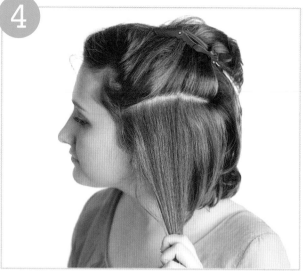

On whichever side of your head your parting is on, divide that section of your hair in half.

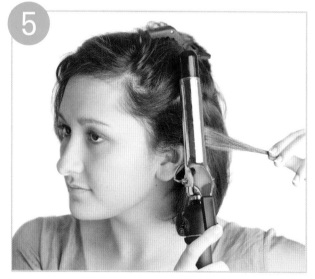

Insert the curling tongs halfway down a piece of hair, holding them open, with the hair at a 90-degree angle from your scalp. Make sure the clamp faces forwards, so you're curling away from your face.

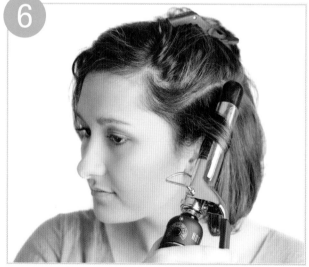

Let the tongs clamp down on your hair, roll them up, then gently glide towards the ends of your hair. Near the ends, loosen tension on the tongs and roll back up towards the roots. Loosen the clamp, bring the tongs almost to the ends, then roll up again.

7

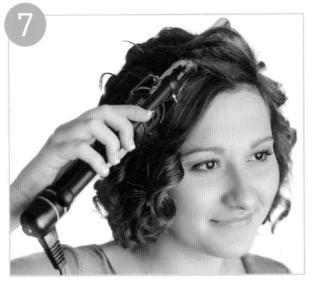

Grab another subsection of hair next to the one you just curled and repeat steps 5 and 6. After you've curled that subsection, release the section above and continue curling.

8

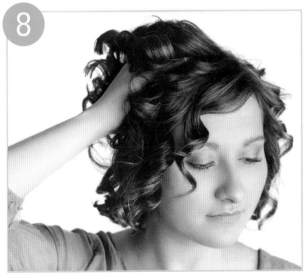

When your entire head is curled and cool, use a defining paste or curling cream to add polish. Squeeze a dollop about 2cm in diameter into your palm and rub your palms together. Work gently through the middle and ends of your hair.

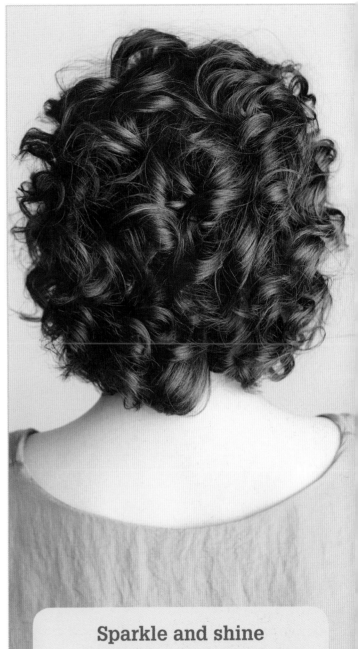

Sparkle and shine

For a little more glamour, spray your curls with a shine spray.

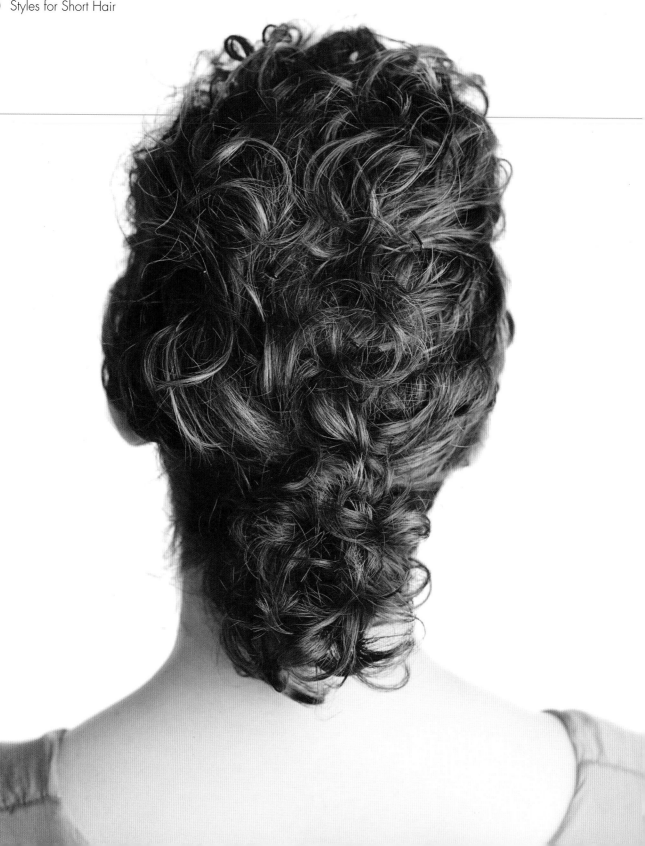

Short and Sassy Pony

SHORT

The ponytail is a deserved classic. Whether you're going for a jog, or getting glammed up for a night out, the simple ponytail can be adapted to suit any occasion. And this shorter, sassier version is equally versatile. The ponytail may be an easy look to achieve, but you don't want to look as though you just rolled out of bed and pulled your hair through a scrunchie. The Short and Sassy Pony transforms the ordinary ponytail into something a bit more special.

TOOLS NEEDED

- hair grips
- clear hair elastics
- sectioning clips
- curling tongs with a 2.5cm barrel
- defining paste
- backcombing comb
- light-hold hairspray

If you have straight or wavy hair, prep your hair with a root-lifting spray for volume at the crown, and a light-hold gel or mousse from the middle to the ends of your hair. If you have curly hair, instead use a conditioning or moisturizing serum on the middle and ends, followed by a holding product, such as a gel or mousse.

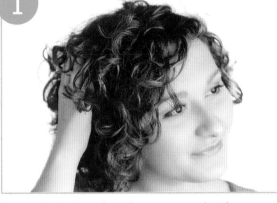

Start with dry hair that's been prepped with a light-hold product.

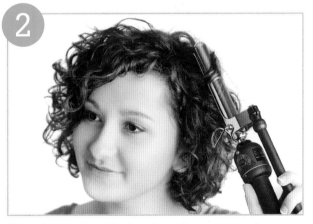

If your hair is shoulder length or shorter, use curling tongs with a 2.5cm barrel to add some texture.

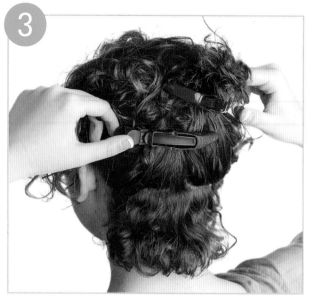

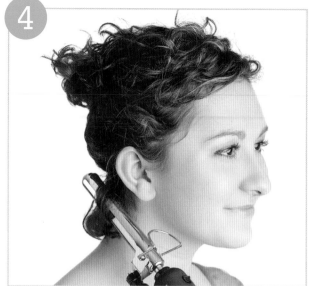

Part your hair where you normally part it. Leave about a 5cm section on the underside of your hair and clip the rest up out of the way.

Use the curling tongs to curl your hair away from your face. Your goal here is not to create perfect tendrils but to add texture and movement to your hair. Make sure you curl all the way to the ends.

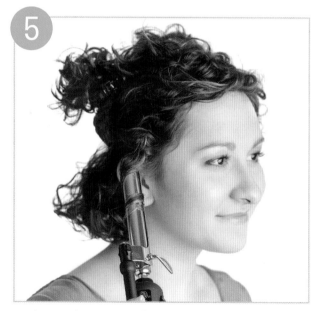

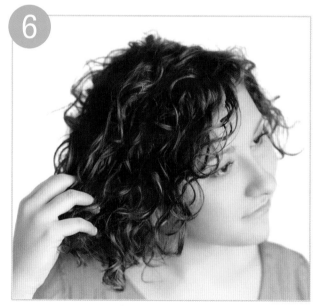

Unclip another section of hair above the section you just curled, and curl the new section away from your face. Repeat until your entire head is full of waves.

Gently rake through the waves with your fingers to soften them.

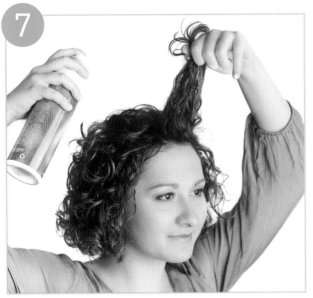

Lift up a portion of hair at your hairline in the fringe area and spray it with a light-hold hairspray.

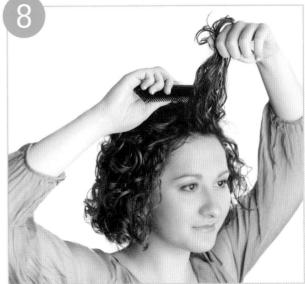

Gently use your backcombing comb to create lift. Repeat, working back towards the top of your head, until you have backcombed the entire crown area.

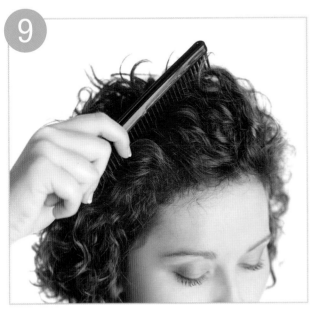

Lightly comb over and smooth the area you just backcombed.

Protecting your hair

Is backcombing bad for your hair? Not if you do it correctly. The key is to use a special backcombing comb, which allows you to create volume without damage.

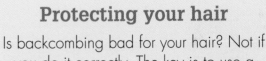

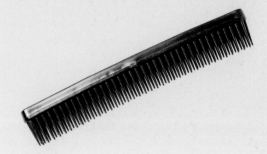

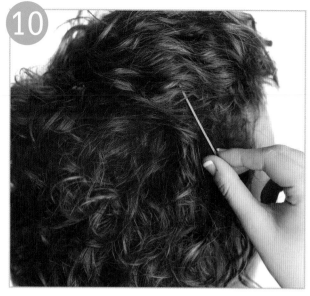

Use hair grips on any loose ends that aren't long enough to reach your ponytail, securing them back and away from your face.

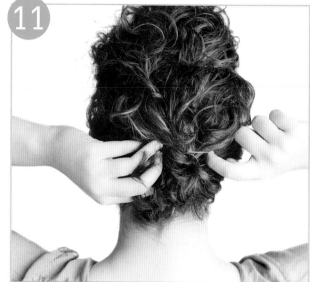

Gather your hair into a medium to low ponytail and secure it with a clear elastic. Your ponytail should look polished but not perfect. A little texture is required for this look.

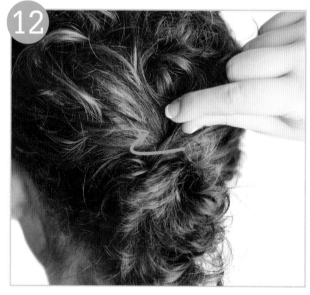

If your hair is long enough, wrap a small section of hair from your ponytail around the elastic, and secure it with a hair grip hidden under your ponytail.

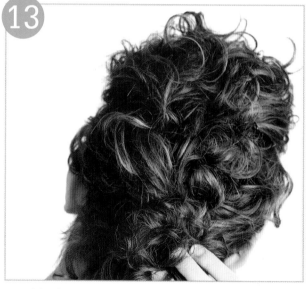

To add additional texture to the ends of your hair, squeeze a dollop of defining paste into your palm. Rub your hands together and then scrunch the paste into your ponytail.

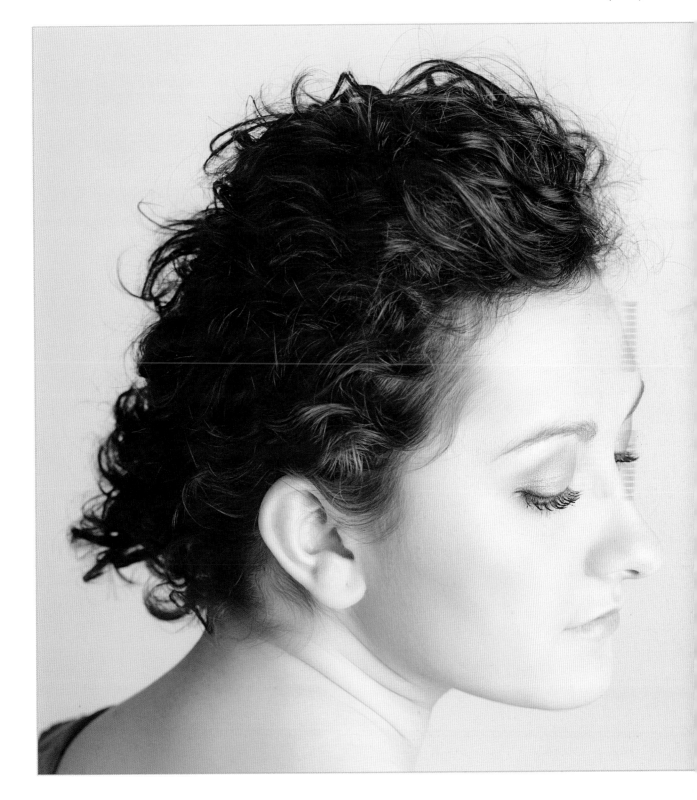

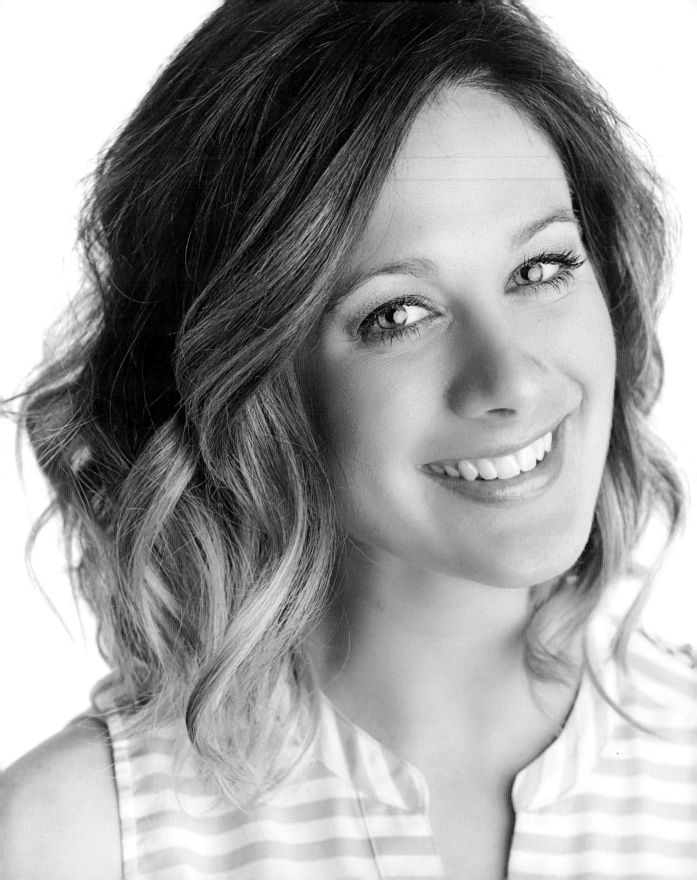

Styles for Medium-Length Hair

Medium-length hair has been making a comeback, starting with the "Lob" or the "Long Bob", which you may have seen on the covers of celebrity magazines. In the past, medium-length hair was all too often thought of as a temporary stage between a short cut and the long hairstyle that you really wanted. So it wasn't always given the most up-to-date styling treatment.

The good news is that times have changed. Exciting medium-length hairstyles are easy to create and offer plenty of options, whether you want a casual look for a walk in the countryside, or need a dressed-up hairdo for a night on the town. These up-to-date styles will have you loving your mid-length hair – and make lingering long-hair envy a thing of the past.

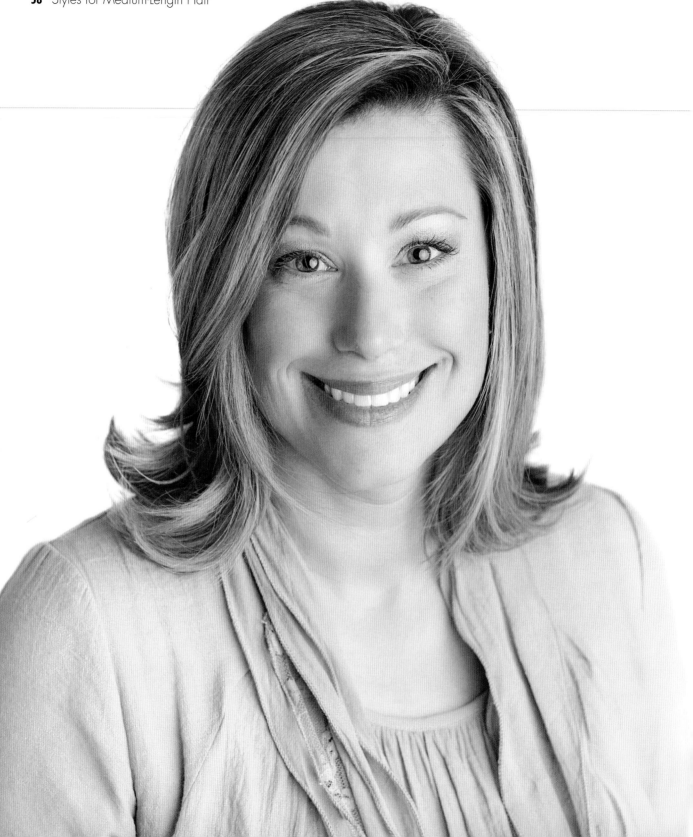

Flipped Out

MEDIUM

This fun style lets you get creative with your hair, with the top portion turned under and the bottom section flipped up. The turned-up hairstyle is a great way to reinvigorate your style for a workday or an afternoon out shopping with the girls. Most hair types will find this style easy to achieve. If you are blessed with a little bit of natural wave, your tresses may stay "flipped" a bit longer.

Fine to medium hair types should begin with a root-lifting spray and volumizing mousse. For thick hair, use a combination of moisturizing serum with a light-hold gel or mousse.

TOOLS NEEDED

- sectioning clips
- hairdryer
- concentrator nozzle
- light-hold defining paste
- paddle brush
- root booster
- round brush (the smaller the size, the more curl at the bottom)
- sculpting lotion
- volumizing mousse

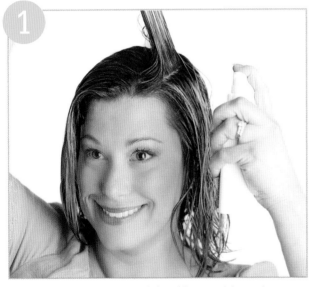

Start with thoroughly towel-dried hair. Add a volumizing mousse and/or sculpting lotion, with some root booster for extra body.

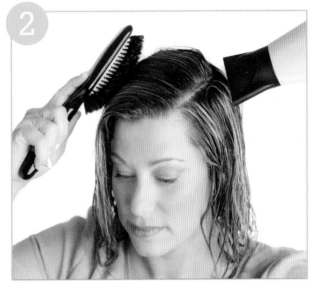

Using your hairdryer with a concentrator nozzle attached, paddle brush your hair, moving in opposite directions, to smooth and tame your tresses.

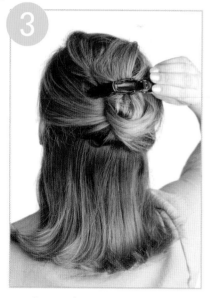

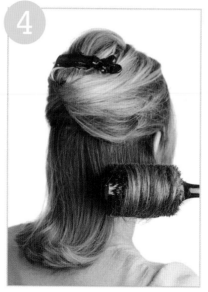

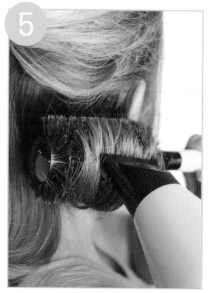

Divide your hair into two sections, one on top and one at the bottom. Clip the top section up out of your way.

Push your round brush on the top of the bottom section of hair, while rolling the brush upwards.

Rotate the brush when you reach the ends, keeping the hairdryer blowing from the roots to the ends.

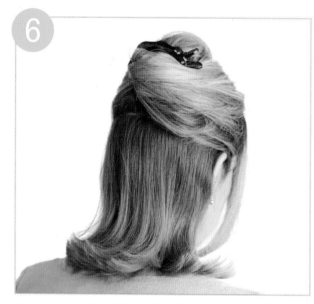

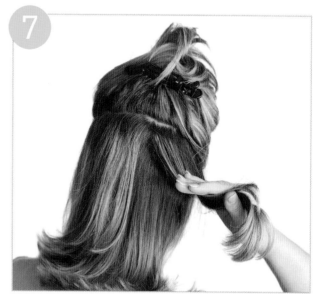

Repeat steps 4 and 5 until the bottom section of your hair is all flipping upwards.

Release a horizontal subsection from the top, clipped-up section of hair, and let it rest just above the flipped-out pieces underneath.

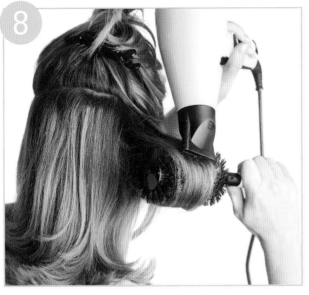

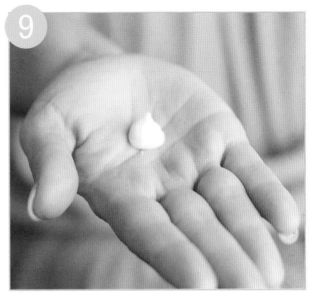

Round brush this section to curl under. Make sure you create tension with the round brush while using the concentrator nozzle, and rotate a few times at the ends of your hair for extra bounce. Unclip and repeat with the rest of your hair.

To finish, squeeze a dollop about 2cm in diameter of light-hold defining paste into your palm. Distribute the paste by rubbing it in your hands before applying through your hair. This creates flow, and separates the style into body-boosting pieces for more volume and movement.

Drying with care

Never blow hot air up the hair shaft. This can cause major frizz and damage.

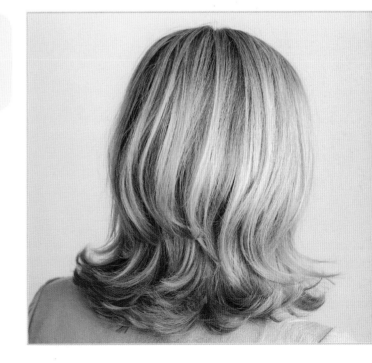

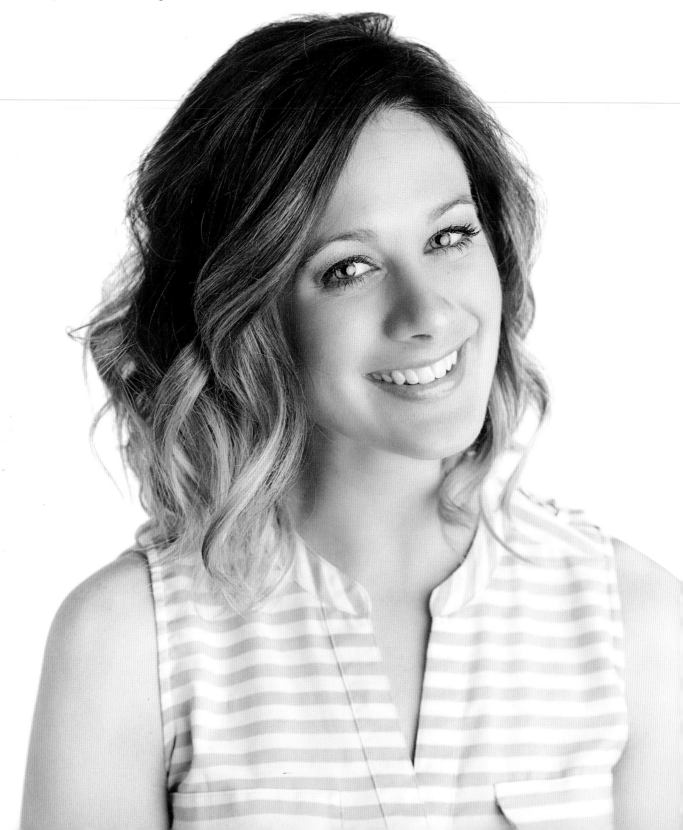

Beach Waves

MEDIUM

This hairstyle looks like you spent the day at the beach, basking in the sun and splashing around in the water. These beach-worthy waves are a bit polished, yet still give a relaxed, slightly tousled and undone appearance.

You can wear these waves casually or dress them up with a hair accessory for an evening out. This look is suitable for longer lengths too, and it's great with all textures of hair. Curly- or wavy-haired girls can work with their natural texture and add polish, whereas anyone with straight hair can achieve this look with a little help from some large-barrel curling tongs.

TOOLS NEEDED

- sectioning clips
- curling tongs with a 3cm barrel
- defining paste
- hairpins (optional)
- light-hold hairspray (optional)
- sea-salt spray
- volumizing mousse

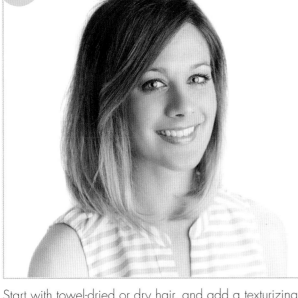

Start with towel-dried or dry hair, and add a texturizing product, such as a sea-salt spray or volumizing mousse. For curly or wavy hair textures, let hair dry naturally.

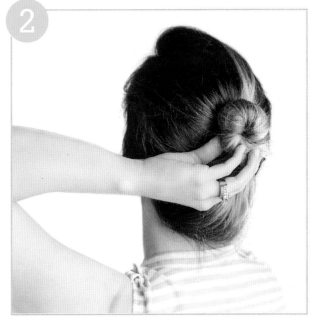

If you have straight hair, you can create a bit of texture by adding product, gathering your hair in a high messy bun, securing it with hairpins, and letting it dry.

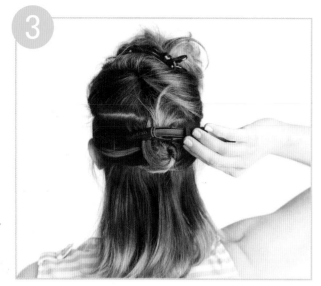

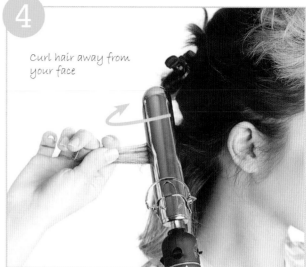

Curl hair away from your face

After your hair is completely dry, and has some texture, separate it into three horizontal sections. Clip up the top two sections, and leave the bottom section down.

Starting closest to your face, hold a 2.5 to 5cm section of hair at the ends with your fingers. With the clamp of the curling tongs facing forwards, open them and place your hair between the barrel and the clamp, at the centre of the section of hair. Close the clamp, and curl your hair away from your face.

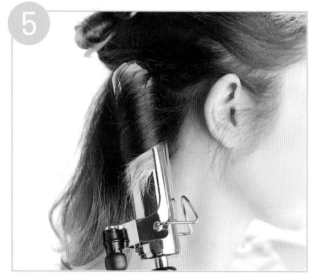

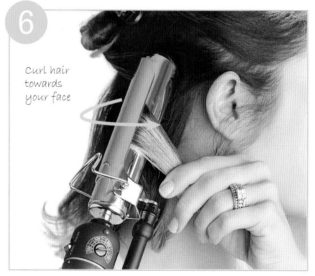

Curl hair towards your face

After you've curled the section close to your scalp, release the clamp of the curling tongs to let a little hair slide out, until about 1.25cm of hair is left at the end. Close the clamp, curl back up close to your scalp, and hold for 6 to 8 seconds.

Pick up the next piece of hair, and curl towards your face, using the same technique as in steps 4 and 5, but now in the opposite direction. Repeat, curling in alternate directions, until all three sections of your hair are curled.

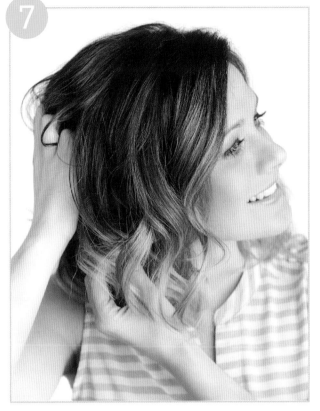

After your whole head has been curled, put a dollop about 2cm to 2.5cm in diameter of a texturizing product, such as a defining paste, in your palms, rub your hands together, and distribute it through your hair in a scrunching motion. This helps comb out the curls, creating a piecey effect.

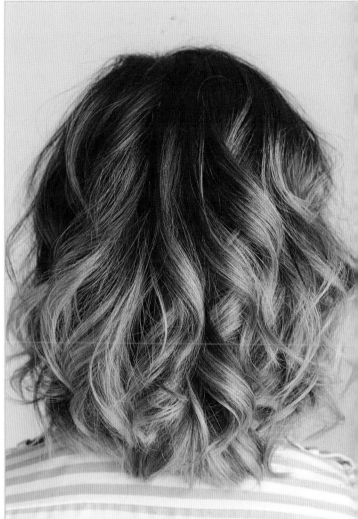

Finishing touches

After you've combed through your hair with your fingers, you can spritz the sea-salt spray on your hair again for an extra-tousled effect. For a more polished look, finish with a light-hold hairspray.

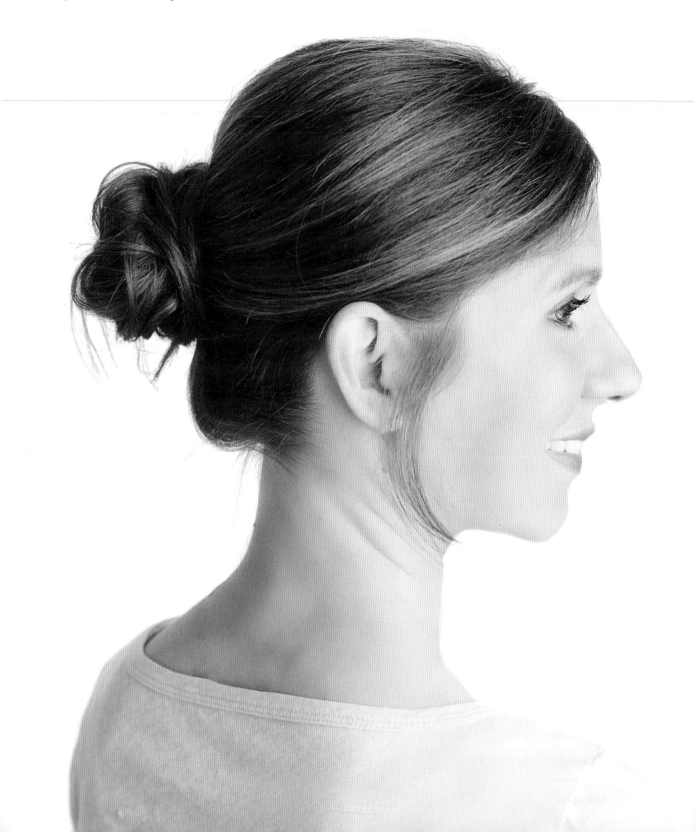

Undone Bun

Anyone with a little texture to their hair will love this fuss-free style. If you don't have any wave, pump up the volume with large-barrel curling tongs. This bun is a quick, chic answer to weekend bed head – and with a deep side parting and pieces loose around your face, easily transfers to the evening.

TOOLS NEEDED

- hair grips
- clear hair elastic
- curling tongs with a 3cm to 3.75cm barrel
- dry shampoo
- backcombing comb

If you've got curly hair, prep with an antifrizz product first and a hold product second. If you have wavy hair, intensify the texture with a sea-salt spray and air-dry your hair for extra oomph. If you have straight strands, use root lifter and volumizing mousse for hold and fullness.

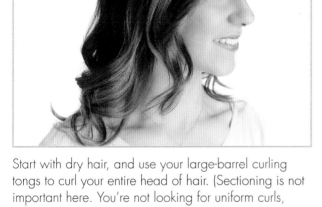

Start with dry hair, and use your large-barrel curling tongs to curl your entire head of hair. (Sectioning is not important here. You're not looking for uniform curls, only texture.)

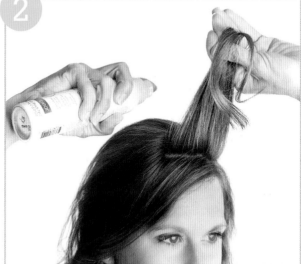

For some additional volume on top, lift up your crown section, spray the hair with a dry shampoo for added texture, and use the backcombing comb to create a little extra volume.

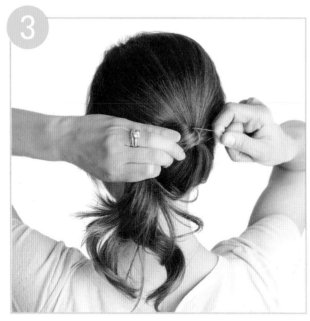

Gather your hair in a medium to low ponytail and secure it with a clear elastic. For extra volume, you could backcomb your ponytail at this point, too.

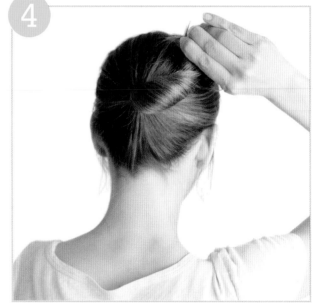

Twist your ponytail until it starts to bend. It will continue to bend round in a circular bun shape as you continue to twist.

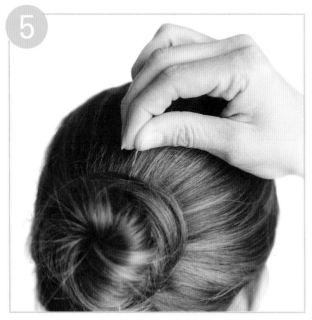

Use hair grips to secure your twisted bun.

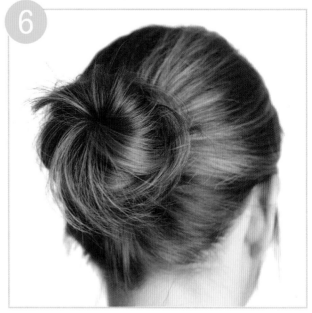

Pull out a few pieces of hair from the bun and tuck them in and around the loop for added messiness.

Texture and style

You can use whatever size curling tongs you like to add texture to your hair in step 1. For medium-length hair, use a wand with a 3cm barrel. If you have longer hair, you can use tongs with a 3.75cm barrel. And remember, for this style your goal isn't to create picture-perfect curls, but to add volume and additional texture.

Give your finished style a retro vibe by wrapping a scarf or bandana around your head to showcase your bun. Or pull your ponytail and, therefore, your bun to one side.

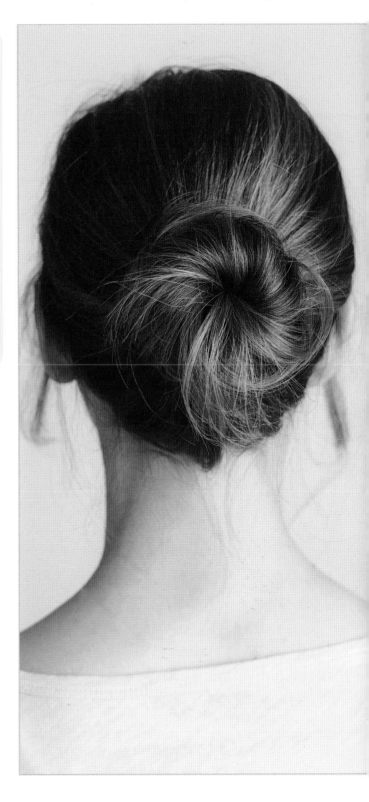

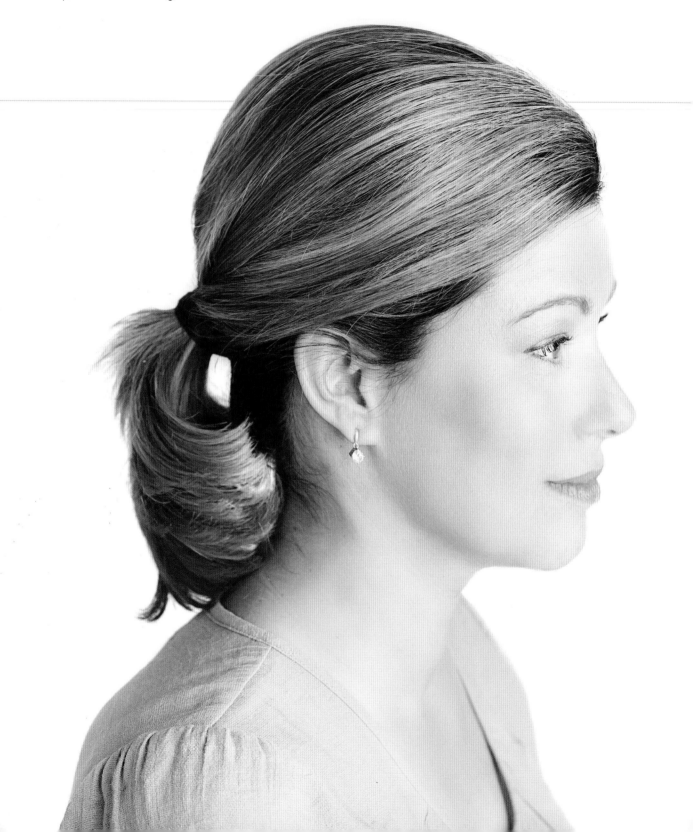

Party Pony

MEDIUM

This isn't your everyday ponytail. The Party Pony is a pumped-up, volumized version of the original. This quick and easy style is great for a girls' night out, a summer concert, or a colleague's birthday party. All types of hair can rock this look; however, wavy and straight hair types will find the style easier to create.

When your hair is dry, you can add extra movement with a wave- or curl-enhancing spray. If you have fine hair, use a dry shampoo to get the necessary volume on the top.

TOOLS NEEDED

- hair grips
- clear hair elastic
- light-hold hairspray or dry shampoo
- backcombing comb

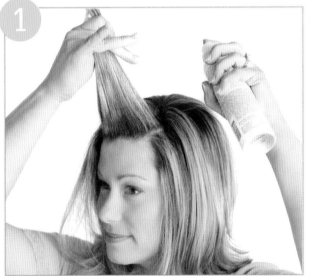

If you have a fringe, lift it upwards and spritz a light-hold hairspray or dry shampoo on the roots for grip.

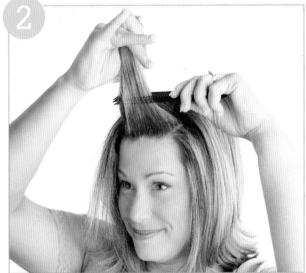

Starting with a 7.5cm to 10cm wide and 2.5cm deep section of hair near your hairline, lift each section of hair upwards and use the backcombing comb in a downwards motion, three or four times. Continue backcombing small sections, moving towards the back of your head, until you reach the crown.

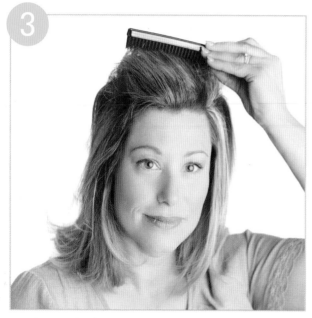

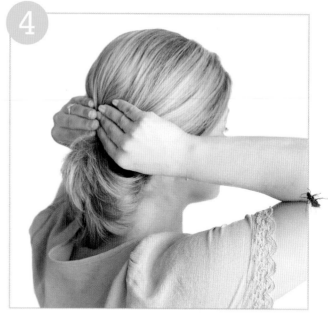

Comb over the backcombed area to smooth the hair and push it back away from your face.

Gather your hair in a high or low ponytail, being gentle with the top section, so it retains plenty of volume. Secure the ponytail with a clear elastic.

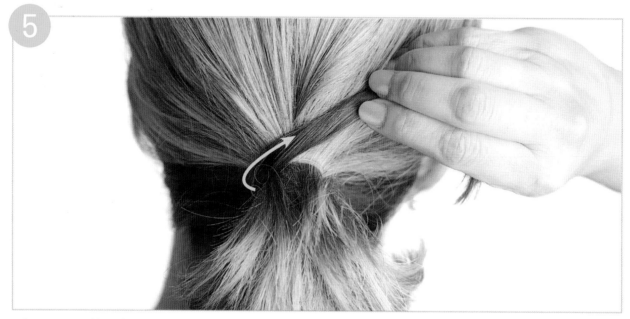

Take a piece of hair from your ponytail and wrap it around to cover the elastic. Use a hairgrip to secure this piece of hair underneath your ponytail.

Adapting the look

You can use a tail comb to create volume and added texture. Insert the comb in your backcombed crown and pull upwards with the end of the comb.

If you have curly or wavy hair, you can also try this style with straight hair. Use hair straighteners before step 1, and you'll achieve a sleek and straight pony.

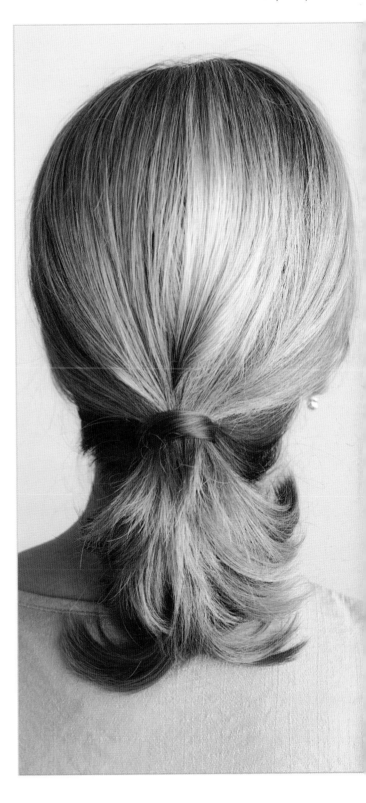

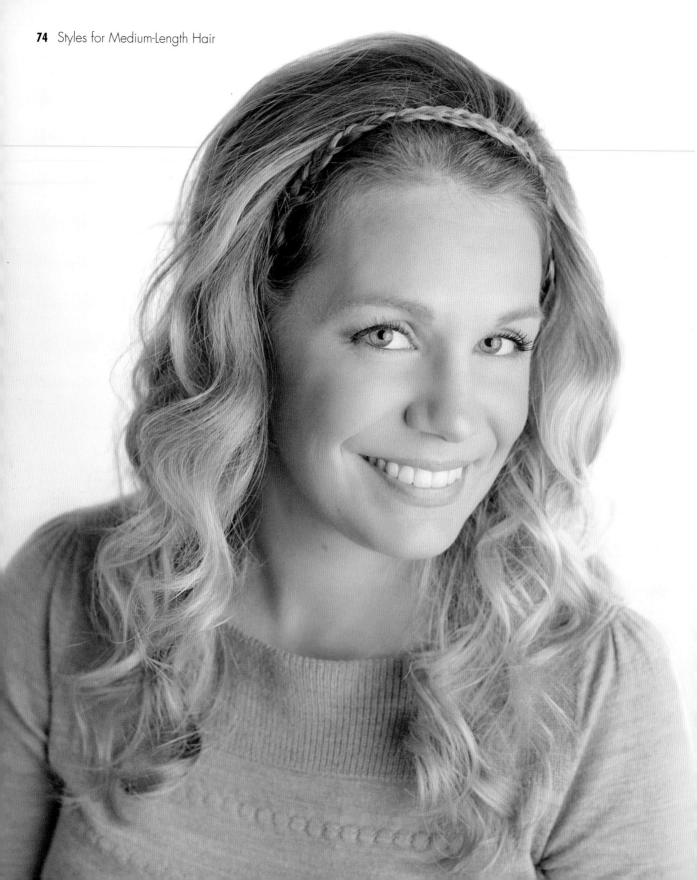

Plaited Headband

MEDIUM

If you're not quite ready to get a fringe, but you still want to try something different, this style is a great choice. The Plaited Headband is a casual style that you could wear for a morning at the gym, but just as easily dress it up for a night out.

You'll need at least shoulder-length hair to get a solid headband. All hair types can achieve this look.

TOOLS NEEDED

- hair grips
- clear hair elastics
- sectioning clips
- backcombing comb

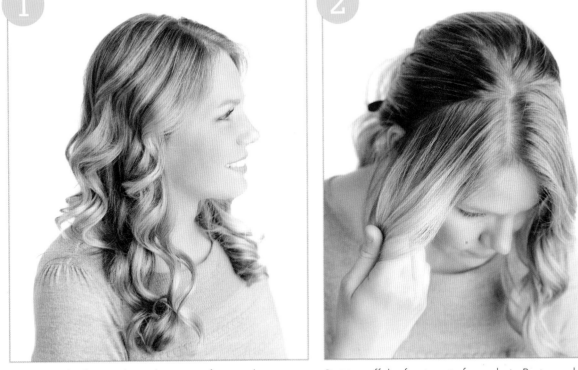

1 Start with dry hair in the style you prefer – curly, wavy, or straight.

2 Section off the front part of your hair. Part your hair across your head from the top of one ear to the other, and clip the rest out of the way.

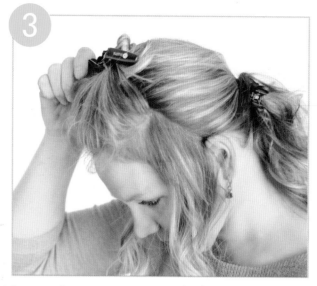

Part your hair again, separating the front section of the hair that is left down. This section should extend from the arch of your left eyebrow to the arch of your right. Fasten this section back with a clip or clear elastic. You should now have two sections of hair hanging down.

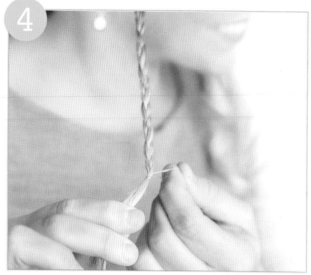

Working with the section of hair on the right, plait it down to the bottom and secure the plait at the end with a clear elastic.

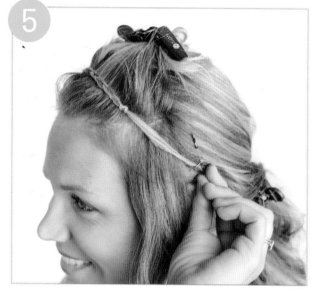

Wrap the plait you have just completed up and across the front of your hair, about 2.5cm back from your hairline. Secure this plait with hair grips to hold it in place.

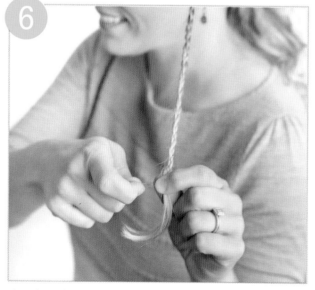

Plait the left section of hair just as you did with the right, and wrap the second plait up and across your head, behind the first, creating a double plaited headband.

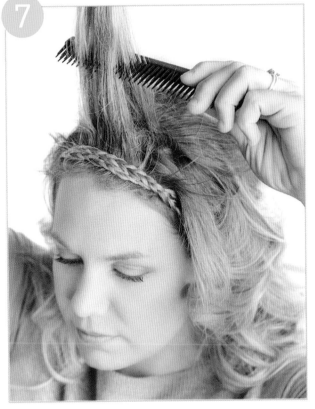

Let all your hair down except for the plaits. You can use a backcombing comb to add some extra volume to the crown section, just behind your plaited headband.

Add a twist

Instead of using plaits, you could twist the lower sections of hair and wrap the twists around your head. Pin these in the same way as the plaits to secure.

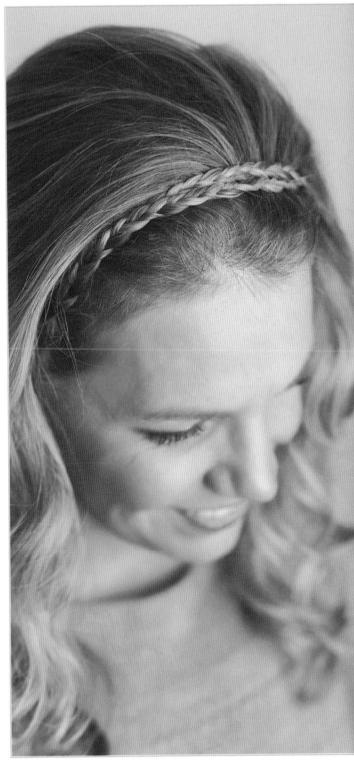

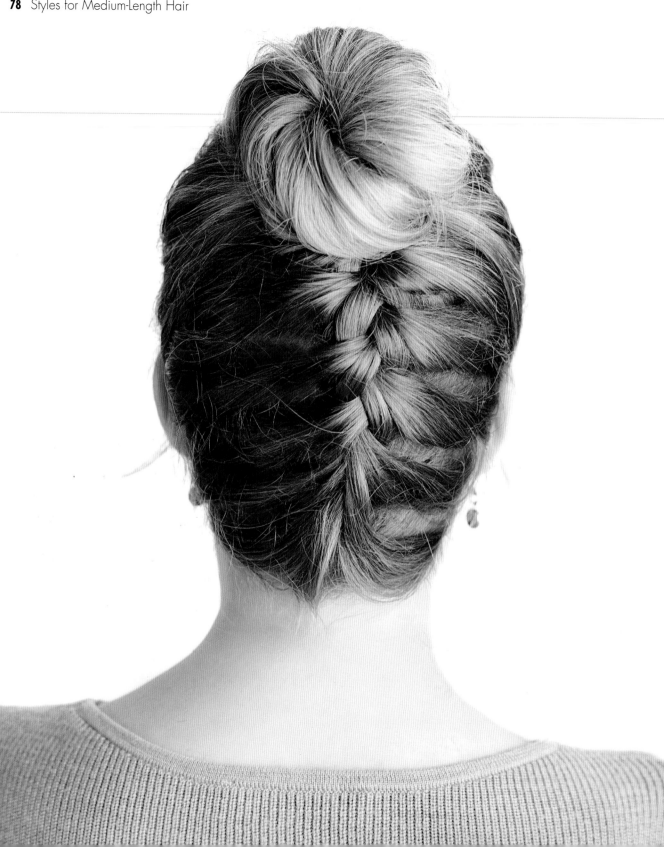

Upside-Down Plaited Knot   MEDIUM

If your ballerina bun needs an update, this style is for you. It's a funky, fresh version of the topknot or plaited bun, and you can wear it just about anywhere. For an extra flourish, you could add a ribbon or other hair accessory beneath the knot. All hair types can achieve this style.

TOOLS NEEDED

- clear hair elastics
- sectioning clips
- hairpins
- medium- to firm-hold hairspray

You want some texture in your hair before you start this style. Slightly curly or wavy hair is best. If you have extremely curly locks, soften and smooth your hair a bit before beginning.

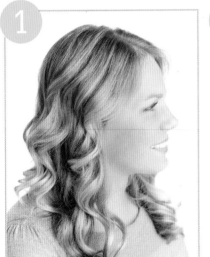

Start with dry hair.

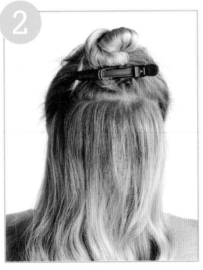

Divide your hair into two sections, parting it from ear to ear. Clip up the top section to keep it out of the way.

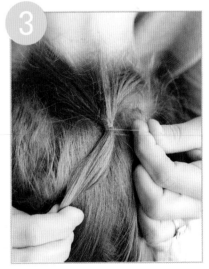

Tilt your head in an upside-down position. Grab a small section of hair at the nape of your neck to begin the French plait. To make it easier to manage, you can secure this section with a clear elastic.

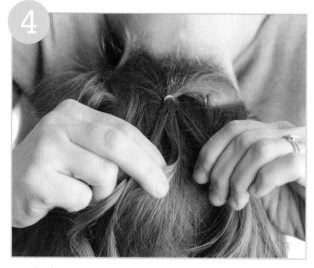

Divide the small section into three subsections.

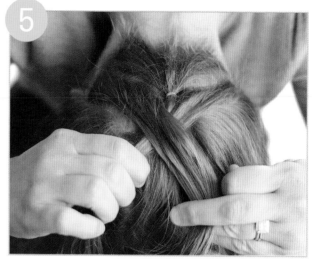

Fold the right side of the subsection over the centre, adding in a small amount of hair from the bottom right. Then fold the left side over the centre with hair from the bottom left, keeping the three sections separate.

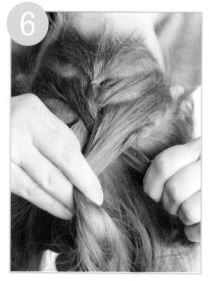

Grab a small horizontal subsection of hair and add it to the piece that's now on the right side. Fold that section over the centre. Before securing your hair in step 7, you can backcomb the crown area, especially if you have fine hair.

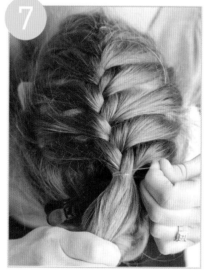

Repeat step 6 for the left side of your hair. Continue the plaiting process until you reach the top of your bottom section of hair. Secure the upside-down French plait with a clear elastic.

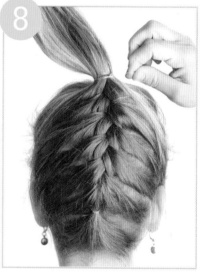

Tilt your head back upright and comb the top section of your hair back to meet the French plait. Combine the two sections into a high ponytail and secure with another clear elastic.

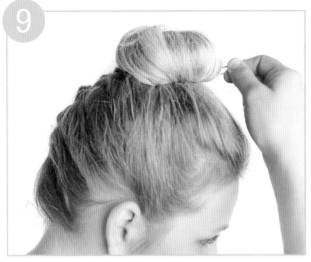

Lift upwards on the ponytail and give it a slight twist. Wrap the ponytail around the clear elastic, into a soft bun, and secure with hairpins.

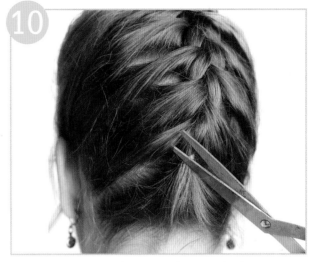

Cut and remove the first clear elastic at the base of your neck.

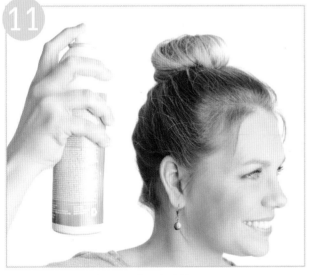

Finish with a medium- to firm-hold hairspray to secure the style.

Pins and bows

To secure your bun with hairpins in step 9, insert a large hairpin into the bun, push it down into the hair beneath the bun and weave it back up into the bun. After you've weaved up and down a few times, gently push the hairpin fully into your hair.

Between steps 8 and 9, you can vary the style by plaiting your ponytail before wrapping it around the clear elastic.

Finally, for an extra bit of glamour, wrap a ribbon around the base of the bun and tie it into a bow at the back.

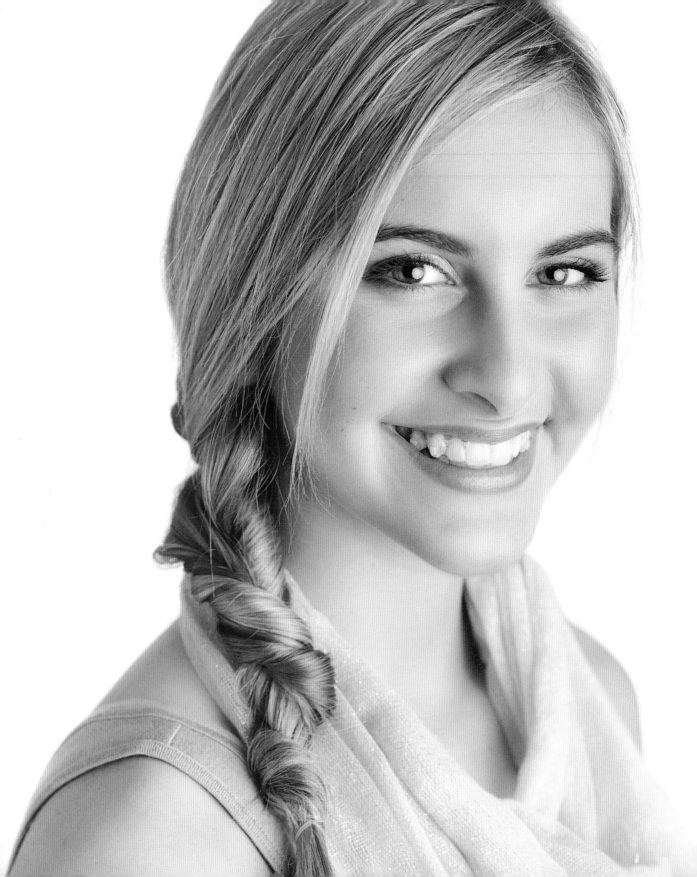

Styles for
Long Hair

Long hair is the most versatile length for styling – it can be plaited, straightened, curled, backcombed, and twisted into an endless variety of styles. Starting with a technique as easy as a basic plait, and leading on to more intricate and eye-catching styles, the step-by-step directions for longer-length styles in this section will have you mastering your long locks in no time.

Tips and tricks throughout will help you to develop your hairstyling know-how, as well as keeping your hair healthy. Trying new looks is more fun when you've grasped the simple steps necessary to bring your hairstyle to life. And once you're confident you've got the hang of the basics, there are more advanced styles to try when you're feeling ambitious.

Long hair isn't hard to style. It's simply a matter of taking the time to patiently work through the steps of each style.

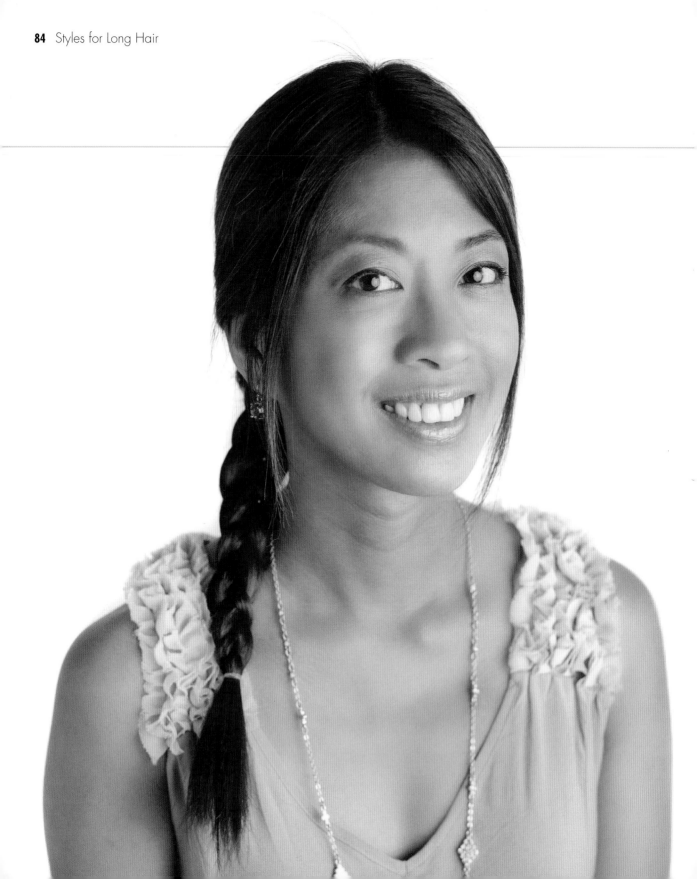

Basic Plait

LONG

The plait is a great hairstyle to learn because it forms the basis of so many other styles. For a stylish but casual look, you can wear a plait low and on one side. Or you can use a plait to camouflage a fringe you're trying to grow out. The plait offers countless simple but sensational variations, and the Basic Plait is versatile enough to wear any time or place. This style is suitable for all hair types.

While you're first learning how to plait, it's best to start this style with dry hair. Once you are comfortable with the technique, you can start it when your hair is damp or wet.

TOOLS NEEDED

- clear hair elastics
- light-hold hairspray

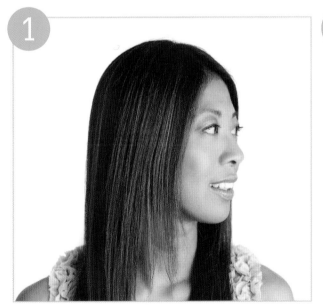

Start with dry straight, wavy, or curly hair.

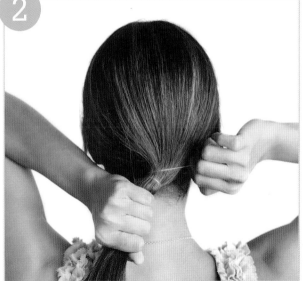

Gather your hair into a low ponytail and secure it with a clear elastic.

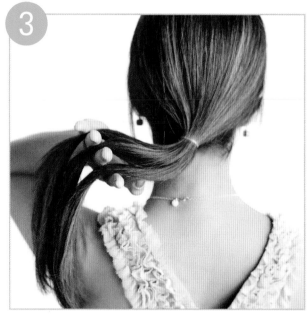

Divide your ponytail into three equal sections.

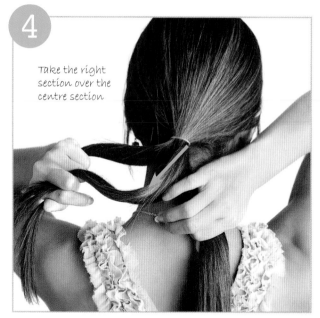

Take the right section over the centre section

Cross the right section of hair over the centre section, retaining the three individual sections.

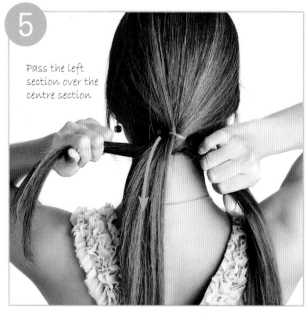

Pass the left section over the centre section

Cross the left section over the centre section. (This is the section that was previously on the right but is now in the centre.) As you get further down, swing your hair over one of your shoulders so that you can see it in the mirror as you work.

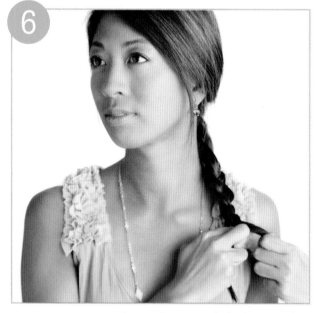

Continue steps 4 and 5 until you reach the bottom of your hair, and secure the end with a clear elastic.

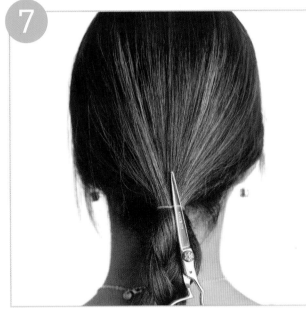

Cut and remove the elastic at the base of your ponytail if you like.

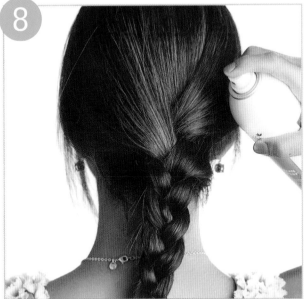

Finish with a light-hold hairspray.

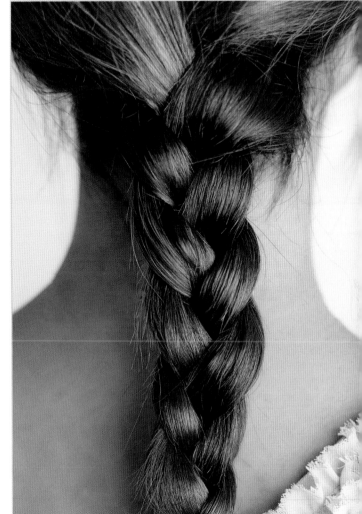

Transforming the look

For quick and easy hair for a night out, backcomb your crown area for a dishevelled look, add a plait, and voilà! You could also curl your hair before braiding to give it a little extra texture, especially if your hair lacks body.

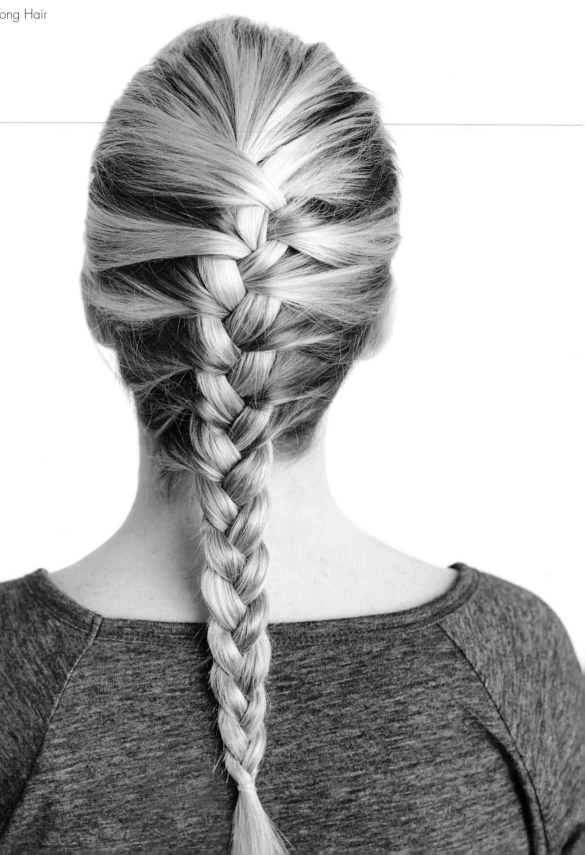

French Plait

LONG

The French Plait is one of those hairstyles that looks harder than it really is. Once you've mastered this style, you can create lots of different versions based on the original design.

This style is easy to dress up or down, depending on how casual you want to go. Straight, wavy, and curly hair all work well with this plait.

TOOLS NEEDED

- clear hair elastics
- paddle brush
- tail comb (optional)

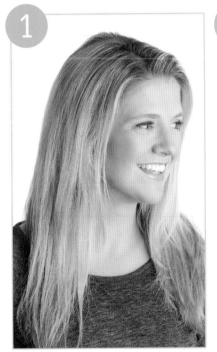

1

Start with dry hair.

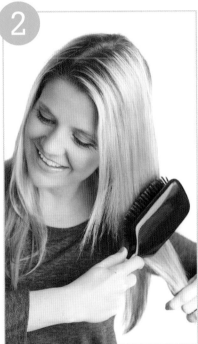

2

Thoroughly brush through your hair with a paddle brush to gently remove any tangles.

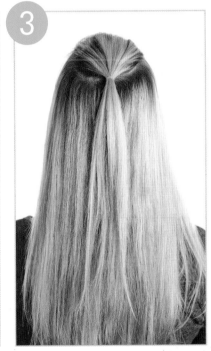

3

Using a tail comb if necessary, part your hair from one top corner of the hairline to the other, in a slight U shape on the top of your head. Gather this section of hair and secure it with a clear hair elastic.

▶

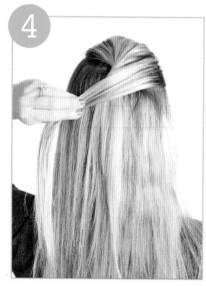

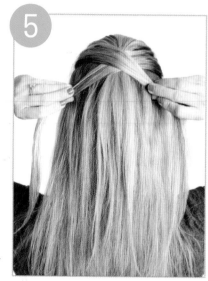

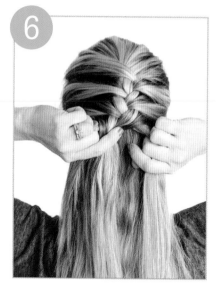

Pick up a horizontal section of hair about 2.5cm to 5cm wide from the right side of your ponytail. Cross this over your central ponytail.

Pick up a horizontal section of hair about 2.5cm to 5cm wide from the left side of your ponytail, and cross that piece over the centre section.

Continue picking up horizontal sections of hair from both sides, working the right section over the centre section, and then working the left section over the centre, as you move down your head.

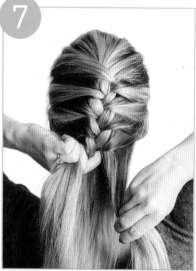

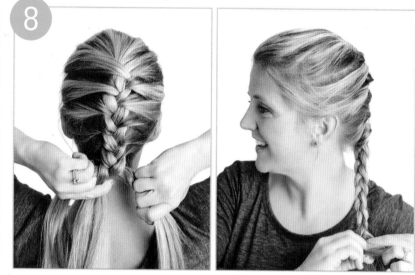

Keep plaiting until you reach the nape of your neck and you have no more horizontal sections to pick up and add in.

Continue plaiting the rest of your hair to the ends. You can swing the plait round to the front to make it easier on your arms as you get towards the end of the plait.

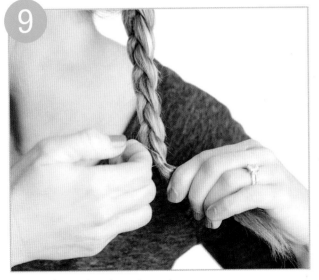

Secure the end with a clear elastic.

A couple of tweaks

You could cover the clear elastic in the top section of your hair, or alternatively cut it with scissors and remove it for a more seamless look.

You also can pull out a few pieces of hair around your hairline for a slightly softer, undone look.

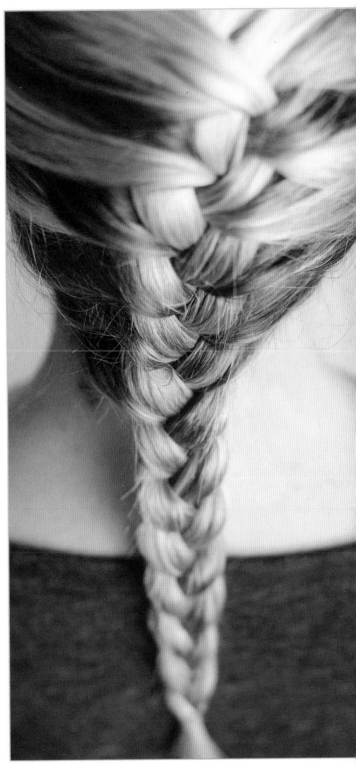

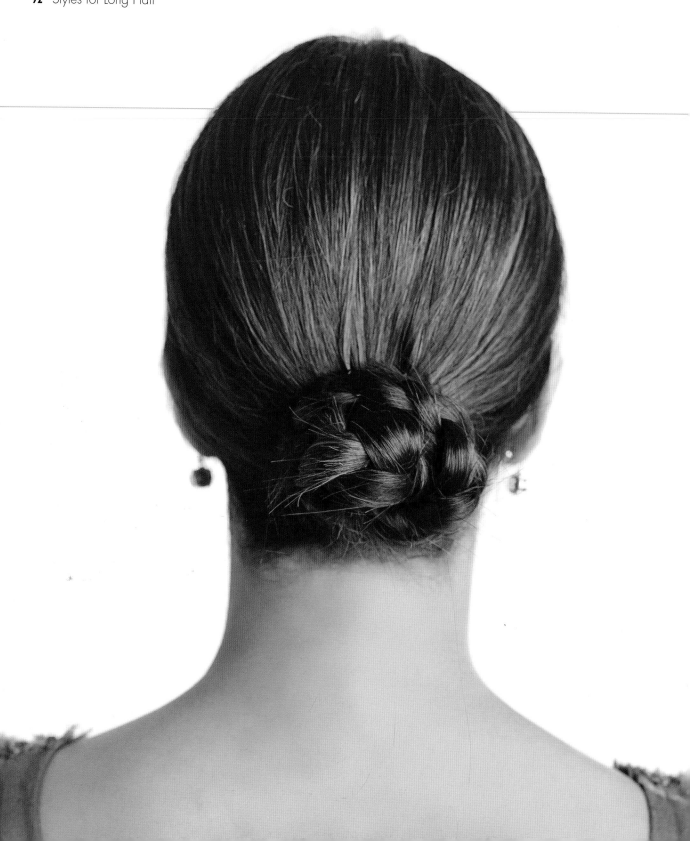

Plaited Bun

LONG

This quick and easy bun has a bit more style than the average bun. You can wear it for a Sunday stroll, tousle it a bit for a sensational runway look, or make it messy for a chic, ethereal feel. All hair types can wear this style.

You can start with any texture of hair for this style. Slightly curled or naturally textured hair will give the best hold.

TOOLS NEEDED

- clear hair elastics
- dry shampoo
- hairpins
- backcombing comb

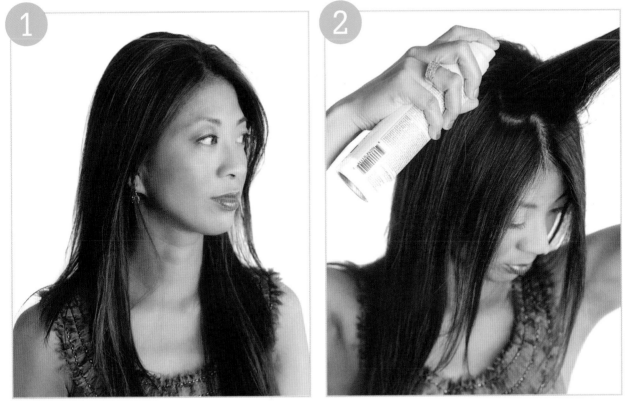

1

Start with dry hair.

2

Grab a section of hair at your crown and spray it with dry shampoo.

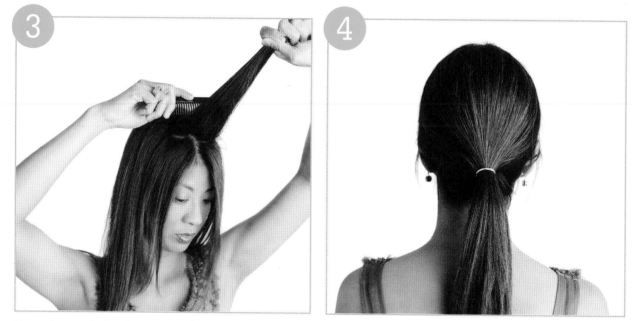

Using the comb, backcomb your crown area for additional texture.

Gather your hair into either a high or low ponytail, depending on your desired look.

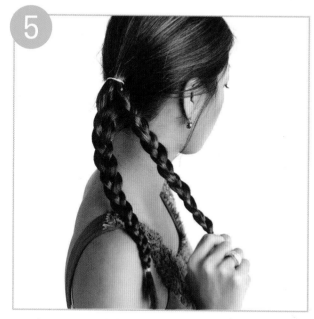

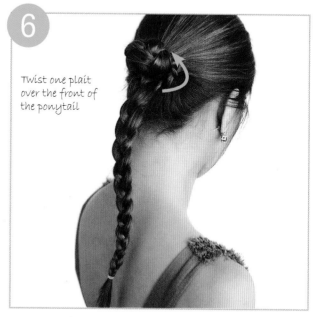

Twist one plait over the front of the ponytail

Divide your ponytail into two sections. Plait each section separately and secure the ends with clear elastics.

Twist one plait around the front part of the ponytail, over the elastic, and secure it with hairpins.

7

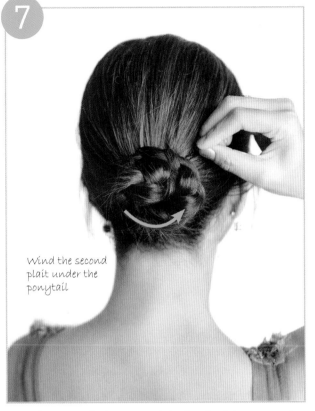

Wind the second plait under the ponytail

Twist the second plait around the back of the ponytail to complete the bun, and secure it with hairpins. Use hairpins to tuck in any additional hairs that are poking out as well.

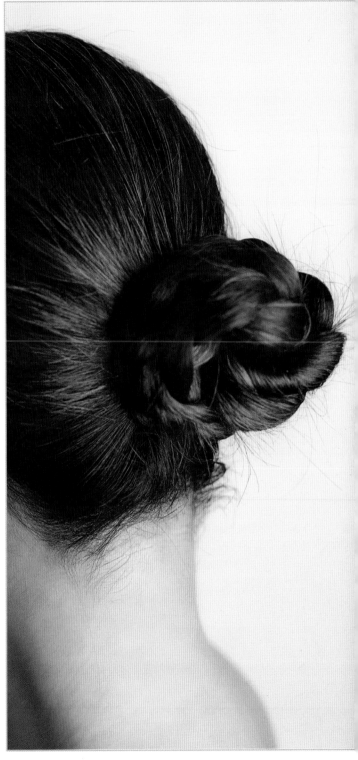

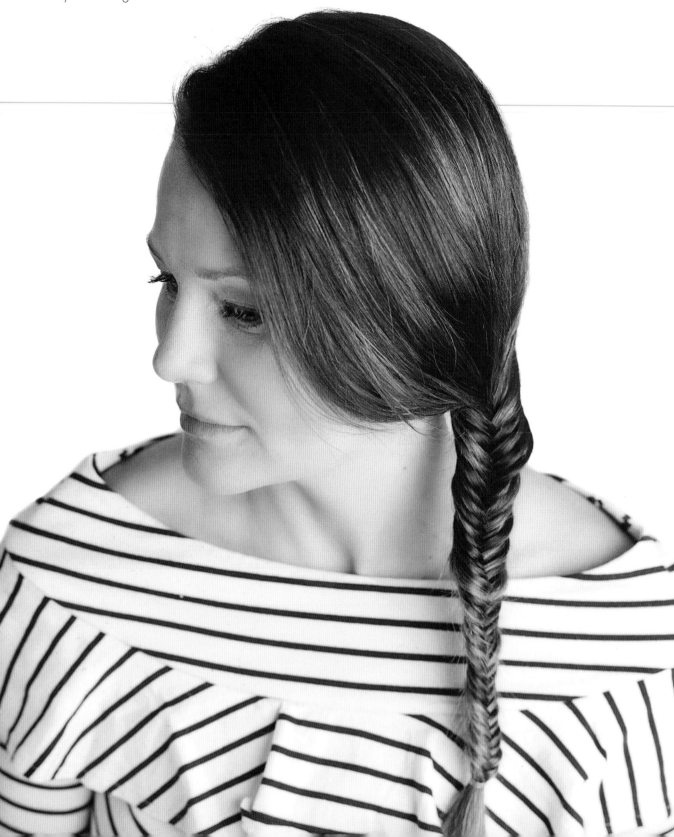

Fishtail

LONG

This fresh new version of the classic plait is making a real splash on the red carpet, but it's also easy to do at home. Wear it to the office, to school, or while running errands. It's a perfect style if you're on the go, because it keeps stray hairs out of your face. Create a polished version for a night out, or a more casual fishtail, with a roughed-up texture and face-framing tendrils. All textures work well with this style.

You can start with any texture of hair. For an undone look, go with a messier texture, and add a spray wax or sea-salt spray. Or you can curl your hair first with large-barrel curling tongs, and then mould your curly locks into the fishtail for a more polished, sophisticated look.

TOOLS NEEDED

- clear hair elastics
- tail comb
- volumizing powder

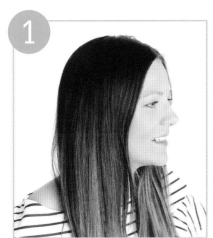

1

Start with dry hair.

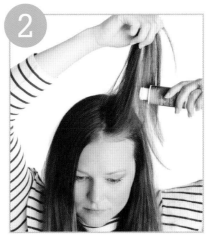

2

Starting in the crown area, sprinkle the roots all over the top of your head with a volumizing powder.

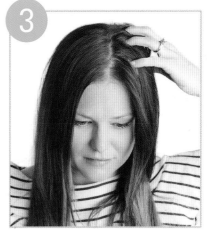

3

Push your fingers into your hair to the scalp where you sprinkled the powder and rub gently back and forth with your fingertips. This helps activate the powder for extra lift. ▶

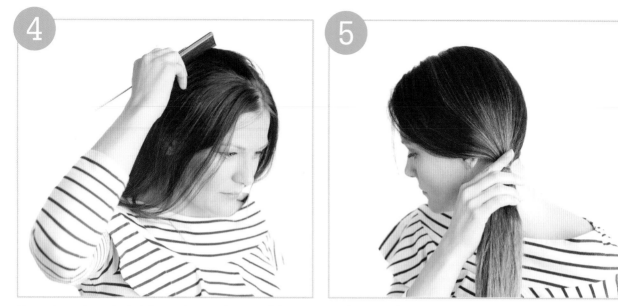

Using the tail comb, lightly comb over the top of the volumized area.

Gather your hair in either a low ponytail or low side ponytail and secure it with a clear elastic.

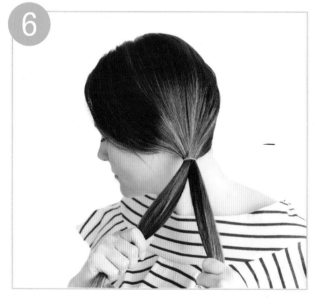

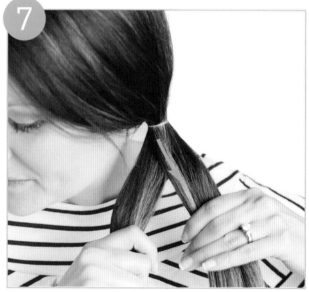

Divide your ponytail into two equal sections.

Grab an outside piece of hair about 3mm to 5mm wide, pull it over the left section, and feed it into the right section. Make sure you keep the two sections of your ponytail separate.

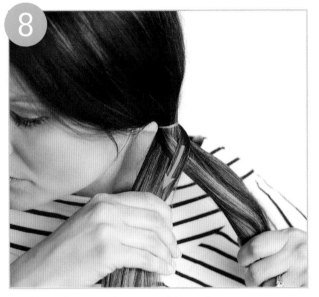

Grab another outside piece of hair about 3mm to 5mm wide, this time on the right side. Pull it over the right section and feed it into the left section.

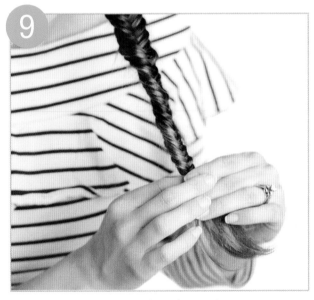

Repeat steps 7 and 8 until you have about 2.5cm to 5cm of hair left unplaited at the bottom, and secure the ends with another clear elastic.

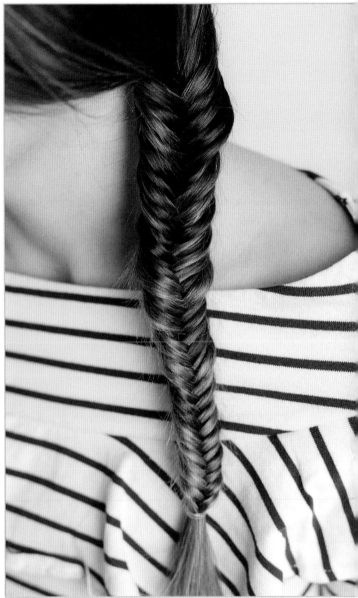

A natural look

To create a more natural flow from your hair into the fishtail, you can cut the first clear elastic you put in at the start of your fishtail.

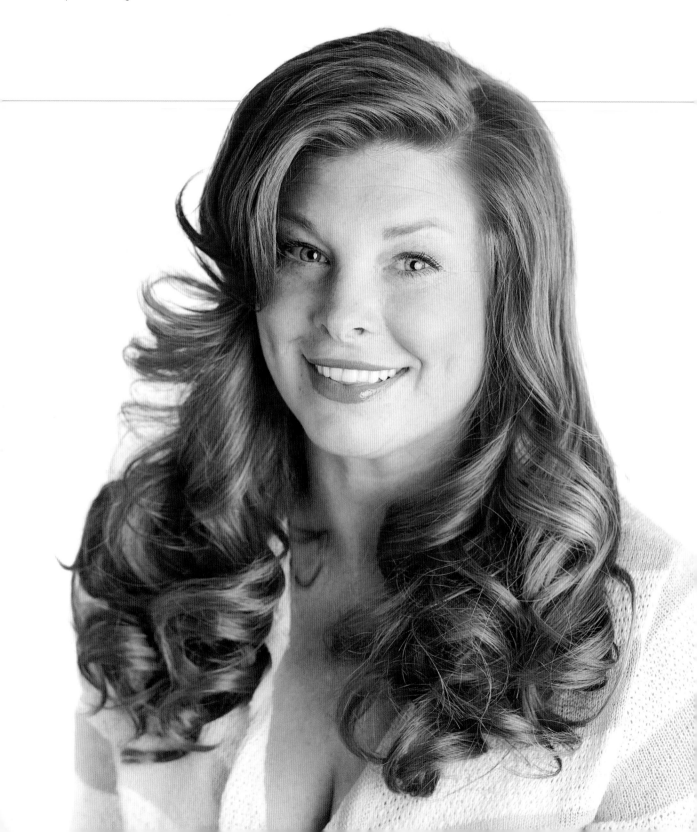

Bombshell Curls

LONG

You'll feel like the life and soul of the party with this gorgeous, classic style. A look this glamorous is best for a night on the town, a friend's wedding, or a red-carpet special event. Although this is one of the more time-consuming styles in the book, because of all the sectioning and clipping you do before curling your hair, the end result is totally worth it. All hair types and textures can try this look.

Although this style works with any hair, if you have curly hair, blow-dry it smooth before attempting this look.

TOOLS NEEDED

- boar bristle brush
- curling tongs with a 3cm barrel
- curl clips
- long sectioning clips
- medium-hold hairspray
- tail comb
- volumizing mousse or light-hold gel

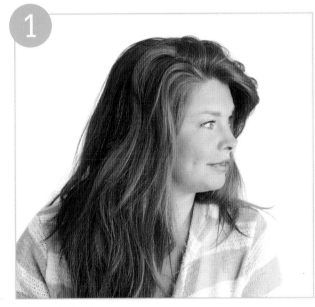

Start with dry hair.

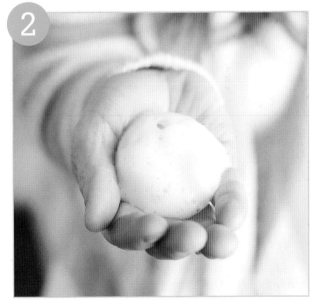

For volume, distribute a dollop about 7.5cm in diameter of a light-hold product, such as a volumizing mousse or light-hold gel, through your hair.

▶

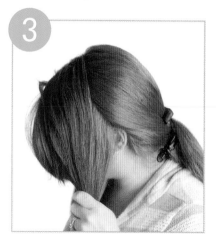

Using a tail comb, divide your hair into two sections, from ear to ear.

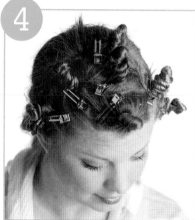

Divide the front section of hair into six or seven 5cm subsections. If you have a fringe, you can section this out separately. Twist each section of hair as you separate it, and pin it with a curl clip to secure it out of the way. Split the back section into horizontal 5cm sections as well.

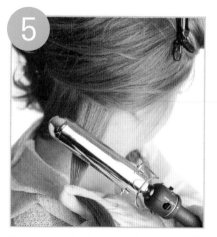

Starting at the bottom of your head, using curling tongs with a 3cm barrel, unclip and wrap a section of hair around the barrel, pointed downwards. Push onto the base of your hair to heat it in the direction you want it to lie.

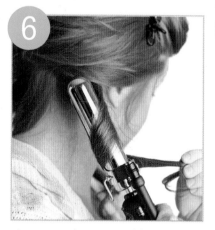

Wrap your hair around the wand so it's flat and not twisted against the barrel.

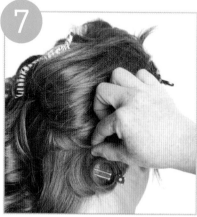

Remove the curling tongs and pin the curl with a clip to set it. Continue unpinning and wrapping sections of hair around the tongs, alternating by curling one section forwards and the next backwards.

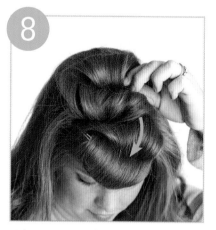

When you reach your top two sections of hair, curl them forwards and not directly on top of your head. You don't want a lot of volume at the crown with this look.

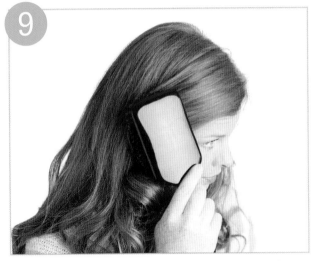

When all your hair is curled, cooled, and set, remove the curl clips and then gently brush your hair with a boar bristle brush.

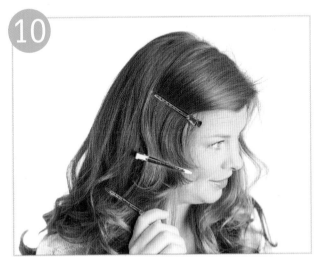

If you need to, you can insert a few longer sectioning clips to help ensure the curls curl the way you want them to and that they will stay in place. Let the clipped curls rest for a bit before removing the clips. Finish with a medium-hold hairspray.

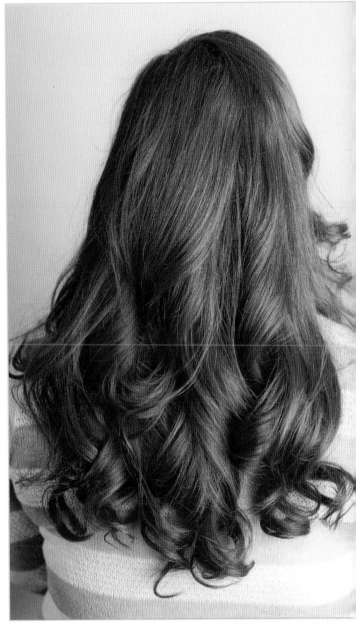

Longer-lasting curls

For extra hold, spritz your clipped curls with a medium-hold hairspray and let them rest for 5 to 10 minutes before unclipping.

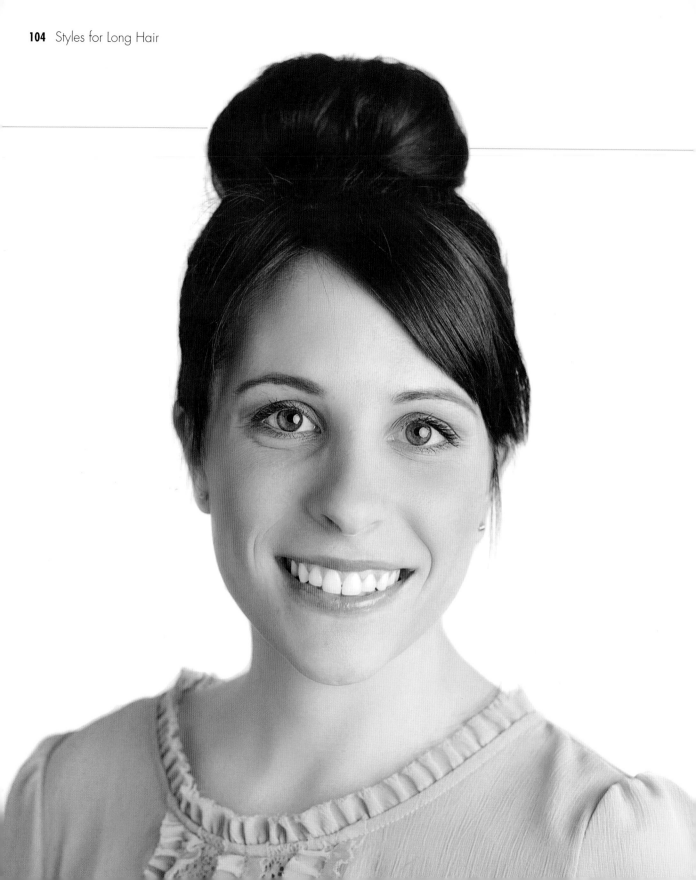

Topknot

LONG

Some days you don't want to spend a lot of time on your hair, but you still want it to look polished. On days like this, the Topknot is your new go-to hairdo. This style is also a great way to disguise second- or third-day hair (washing your hair every day isn't necessarily good for it). It is also a great extender for a blow-dry.

All textures can wear this style, but it works best with straight or wavy hair. You can start with any kind of texture. If you have super-silky locks, for optimal results give your hair some additional texture beforehand, so that the strands will stay better in the bun.

TOOLS NEEDED

- hair grips (optional)
- clear hair elastics
- hairpins
- medium- to firm-hold hairspray
- root-lifting foam
- smoothing serum or paste (optional)
- backcombing comb

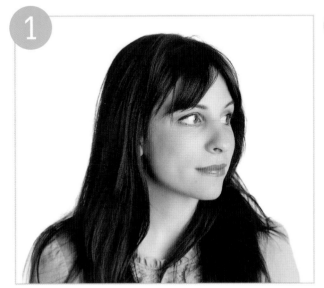

Start with dry hair.

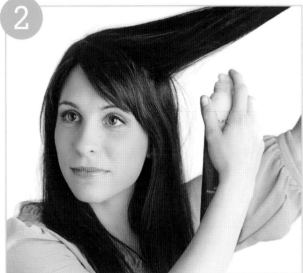

Rough up the texture at your roots by applying a root-lifting foam in the crown area. Do this by separating out long horizontal sections and applying the foam directly to your scalp.

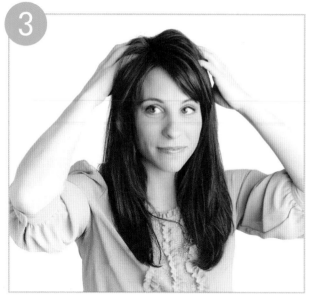

Massage the foam into the roots with your fingertips to create even more texture.

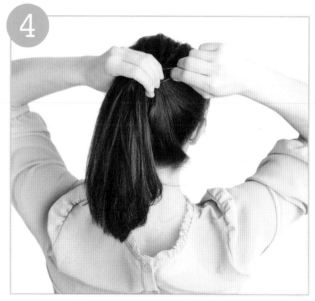

Gather your hair into a high ponytail and secure with a clear elastic. Make sure your pony is free of bumps or knots. You want your hair to look uniform, but not slick and smooth.

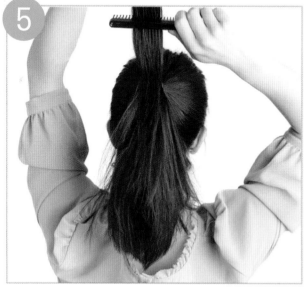

Backcomb your ponytail thoroughly using the comb. This style won't hold unless your hair has plenty of body and texture.

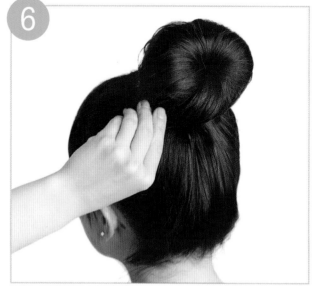

Wrap the ponytail around the front of your head loosely to begin forming the knot.

7

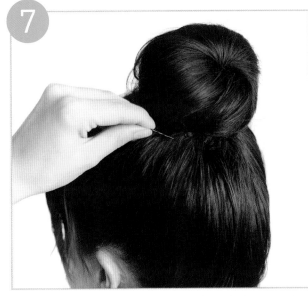

Continue wrapping the ponytail to form the knot until you can tuck the ends underneath. Secure the knot with hairpins and add hair grips if needed for extra stability.

8

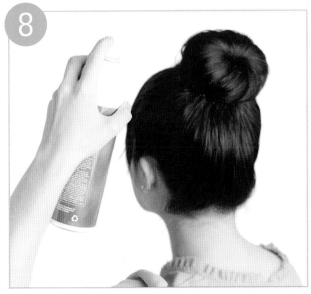

Set your hair with a medium- to firm-hold hairspray. If you have dry or damaged hair, you can use a smoothing serum or paste to help tame frizz and flyaways along the base of the ponytail.

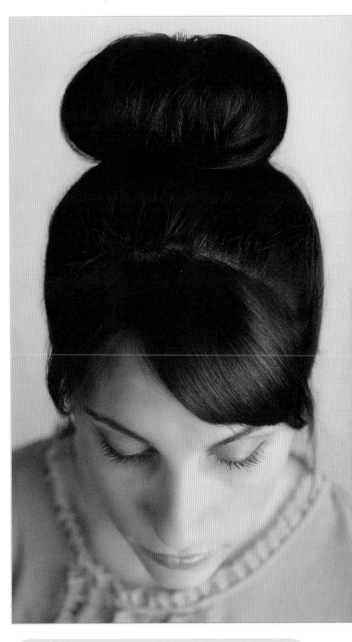

Added detail

Make this style look ultra-modern by placing a bow or decorative barrette directly below the knot on the underside.

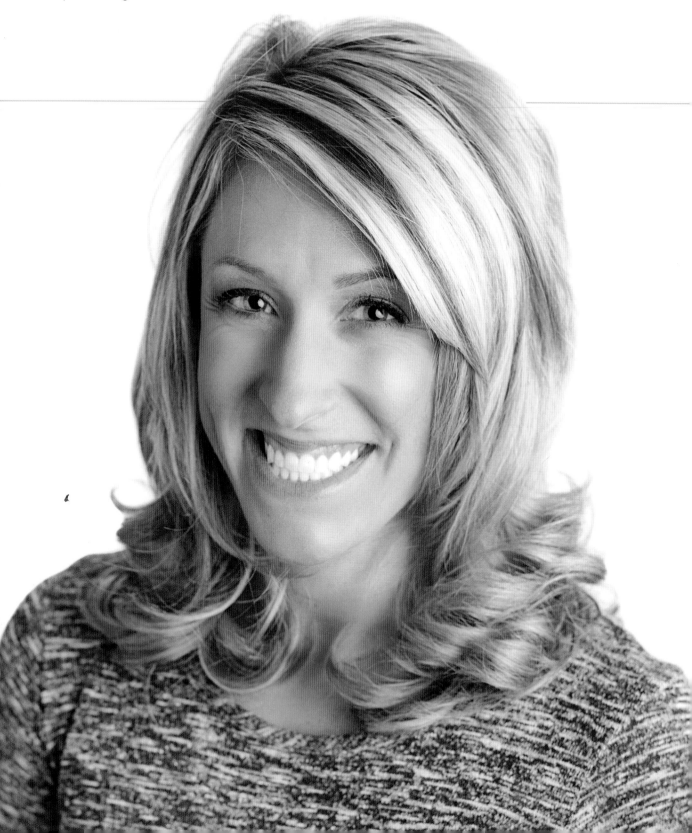

High Roller

LONG

Want luscious curls but don't want to spend a lot of time getting them? Hot rollers are the answer. Not as commonly used as they once were, hot rollers are a simple, time-saving way to get bouncy, voluminous locks. Multitaskers will love that they can put in the rollers, then go and do other things while they cool and curl the hair.

All hair types can use hot rollers. Make sure your rollers are fully heated and ready to go before you put them in your hair. If you have naturally curly hair, especially if it's tightly curled, you might want to blow-dry it straight first before attempting this look. You'll have better luck getting smoother curls if you start with straighter hair.

TOOLS NEEDED

- boar bristle brush
- sectioning clips
- roller clips or flat sectioning clips
- hot rollers
- light-hold curl-enhancing mousse
- light-hold hairspray

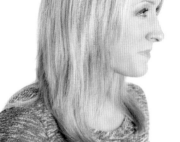

1 Start with dry hair.

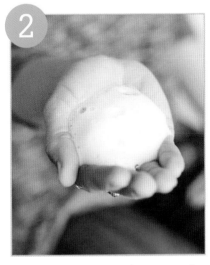

2 Dispense approximately 7.5cm of light-hold curl-enhancing mousse into your palm, for each side of your hair. You want to use just enough to give extra hold.

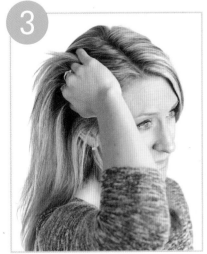

3 Apply the mousse to your hair, working it through to the ends.

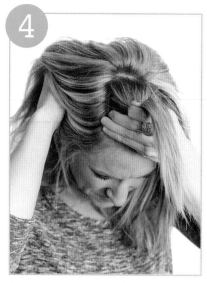

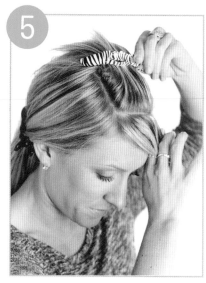

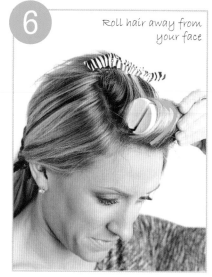

Roll hair away from your face

Section out a strip of hair down the centre of your head (like a Mohican), no wider than the size of a roller. Clip the rest of your hair out of the way.

With your central strip sectioned off, pull out a subsection the length and width of one roller at your hairline. Clip the rest of the Mohican section out of the way.

Pull the section of hair out tight, beyond 90 degrees, and insert a roller, rolling backwards away from your face. Make sure all the section of hair is pulled seamlessly into the roller to avoid any kinks.

Extra volume

Starting by pulling each section of hair out beyond 90 degrees adds extra volume to the finished style. Do this with each section as you roll, for maximum body.

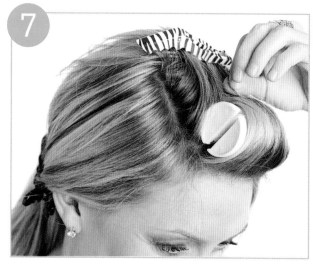

When the roller has reached your scalp and you're ready to secure it, insert a roller clip at the base of your hair, ensuring that you've caught the hair in the roller and the hair at the base to hold it in place while it cools. If needed, insert another clip on the other side.

8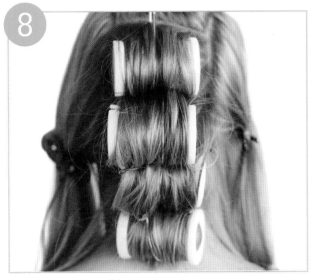

Repeat steps 6 and 7 for the rest of your Mohican section, all the way down to the nape of your neck. Then move to the sides of your head and repeat, sectioning out your hair the width of one roller at a time, until your entire head is full of rollers.

9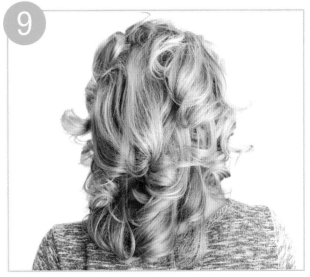

Let the rollers cool for about 20 to 25 minutes. When they're cool, gently remove them.

10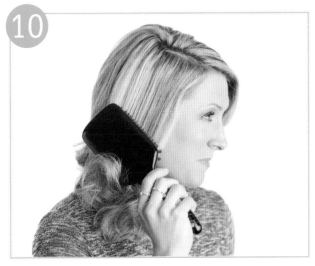

Comb through your hair with your fingers for a tousled, bouncy look, or use a boar bristle brush for a smoother, more polished style. Finish with a light-hold hairspray, so your hair can still move freely.

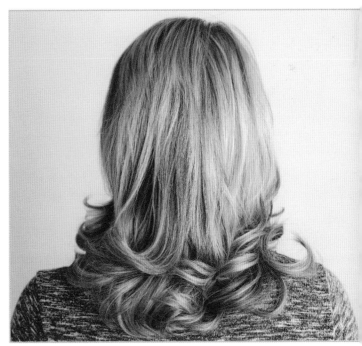

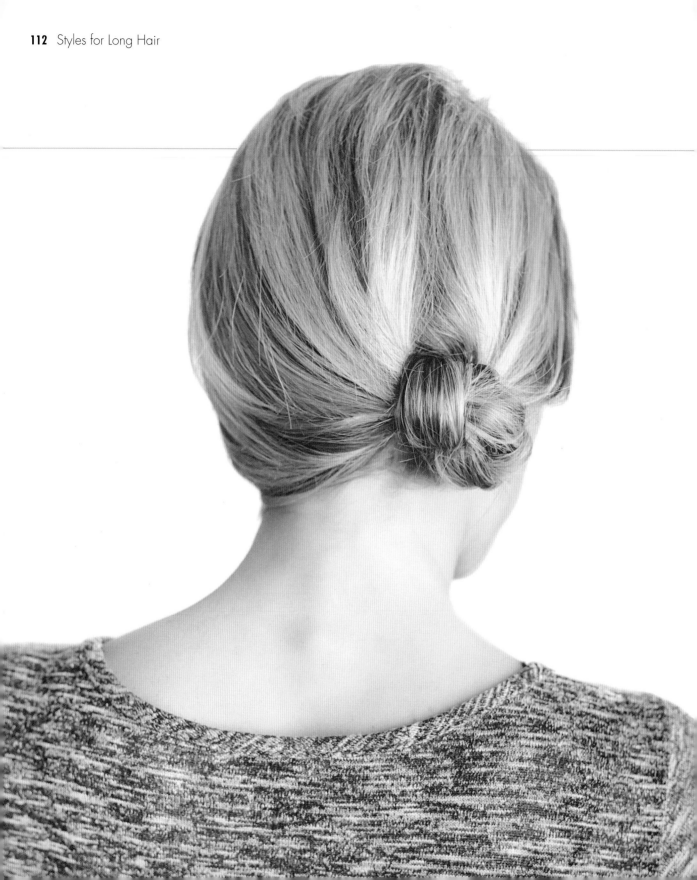

Knot Your Basic Bun

LONG

The basic bun is one of those go-to styles that can be easily dressed up or dressed down for different looks. This version can be formal or casual, too, but whichever direction you take it, it's always eye-catching. In Knot Your Basic Bun, you literally tie your hair in knots. This unique look works brilliantly with all hair types and textures, even extremely curly hair.

For this style, you can start with hair that's been dried naturally, blow-dried straight and sleek, or anything in between.

TOOLS NEEDED

- hair grips and/or hairpins
- clear hair elastics
- hairspray
- backcombing comb (optional)
- volumizing mousse

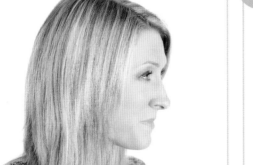

Start with dry hair.

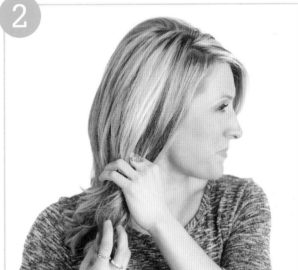

Dispense a 7.5cm dollop of volumizing mousse into your palm. Distribute the mousse by smoothing it between your hands, then apply it to the middle and ends of your hair for additional hold.

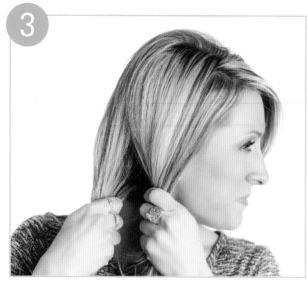

Gather your hair low on one side of your head, and divide it into two equal sections.

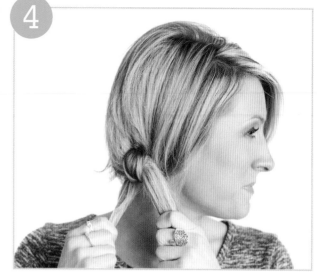

Tie these two sections into a knot, like you would tie the first knot when tying shoelaces. Keep the knot very close to your head, low and at the base.

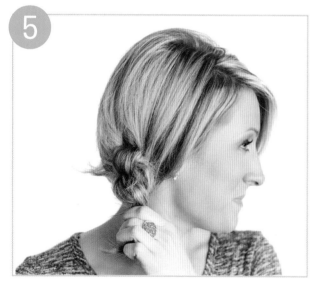

Keeping the first knot taut, tie a second knot the same way just below it.

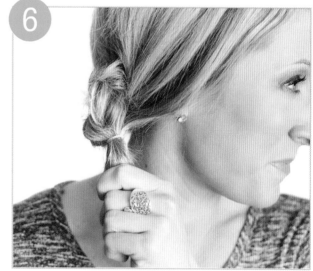

Combine the two tails into one section. Continue to keep the two knots tight at the base of your scalp, and secure the ends into a ponytail using a clear elastic, directly below the second knot.

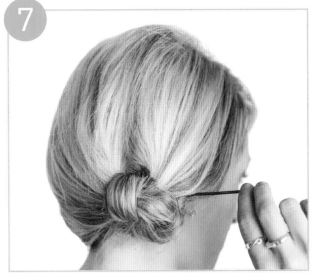

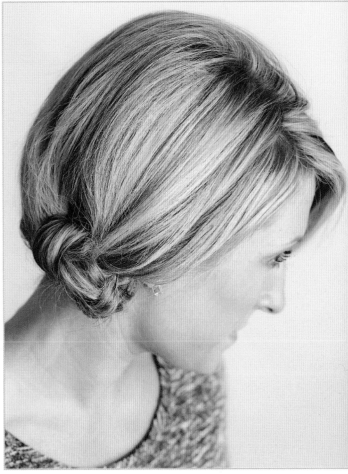

Tuck up the ends of the ponytail to create the bun, and push the elastic up into the second knot to hide it. You can loosen the bottom strand of the second knot a little to cover the elastic better. Use hair grips and/or hairpins to secure the ends.

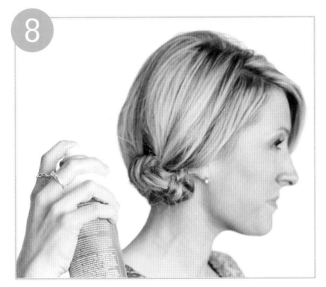

Finish with a veil of hairspray.

Refining the style

If you have short layers, you might need to use hair grips or hairpins on the side of your hair opposite the knot to avoid any flyaways.

If your hair is longer, rather than tucking the ends up into a bun in step 7, you could backcomb to add a little texture to the ends of your ponytail and leave it down. Adding another dollop of mousse to the ponytail will also give increased texture.

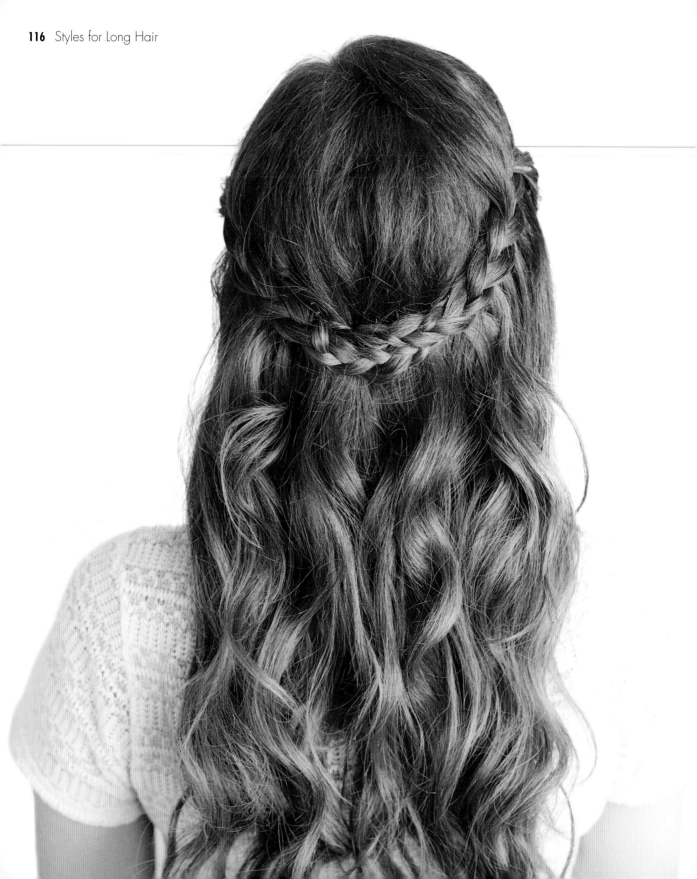

Crown and Glory

LONG

Picture yourself at a summer music festival or picnicking in the park wearing this lovely plaited style. An urban hippie version of half-up hair, it looks like you've put in some effort – but not like you've stood in front of the mirror for hours, adjusting each and every strand. This fuss-free style works well with almost any hair type.

Most hair types can achieve this style, but the more natural texture your hair has, the better your finished Crown and Glory will look.

TOOLS NEEDED

- hair grips and/or hairpins
- clear hair elastics
- sectioning clips
- curling tongs with a 3cm barrel
- defining paste

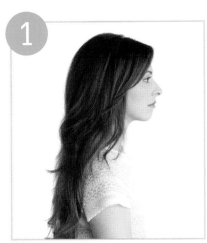

Start with dry hair.

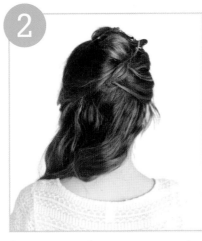

Separate your hair into two equal sections, one on top and one at the bottom, parting from the top of one ear to the top of the other. Clip up the top section.

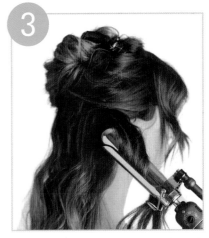

Use curling tongs with a 3cm barrel to add texture to your hair. Starting closest to your face, hold a 5cm section of hair outwards at a 45-degree angle from your head. Insert this section of hair into the open tongs with the clamp facing forwards. Close the clamp in the middle of the section.

▶

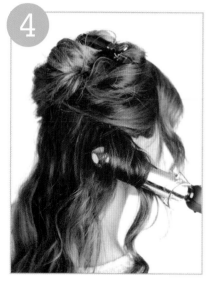

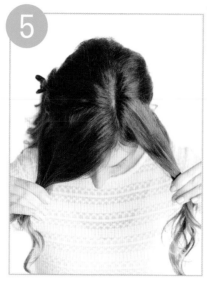

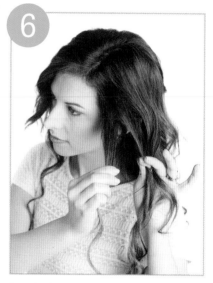

Roll the tongs up towards your scalp. Hold there for 2 or 3 seconds. Continue curling until your entire head is curled.

Separate off a 5cm section of hair along your front hairline and clip it out of the way. Give yourself a centre or side parting.

Divide the section on one side of your parting into three subsections.

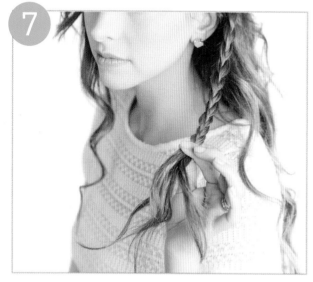

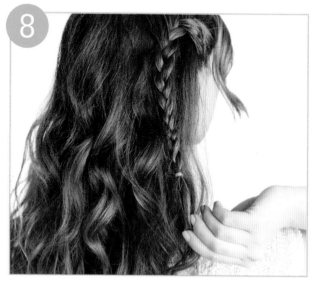

Either French plait for a couple of sections and then transition to a standard plait, or do a standard plait from the start. When you've finished, secure the plait with a clear elastic.

Repeat steps 6 and 7 with the section of hair on the other side of your parting. You now have two plaits.

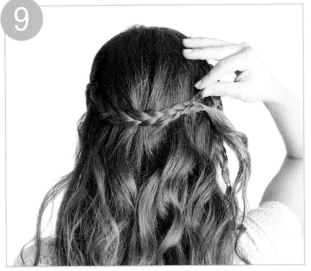

Wrap the right plait loosely behind your head and use hairpins or hair grips to secure it.

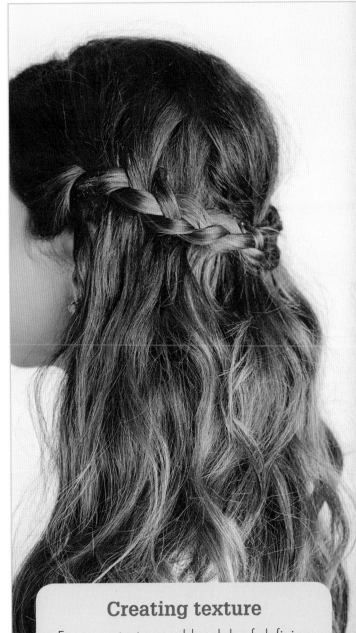

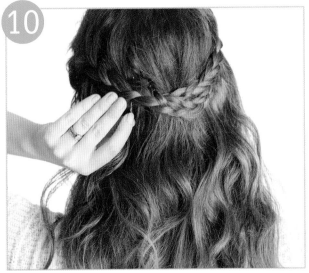

Wrap the left plait behind your head, over the first plait, and tuck it in. Try to hide the elastic under the second plait, and use hair grips wherever necessary to anchor the plaits to your head so they don't move.

Creating texture

For more texture, add a dab of defining paste to your fingertips, then pull out and style some strands around your face.

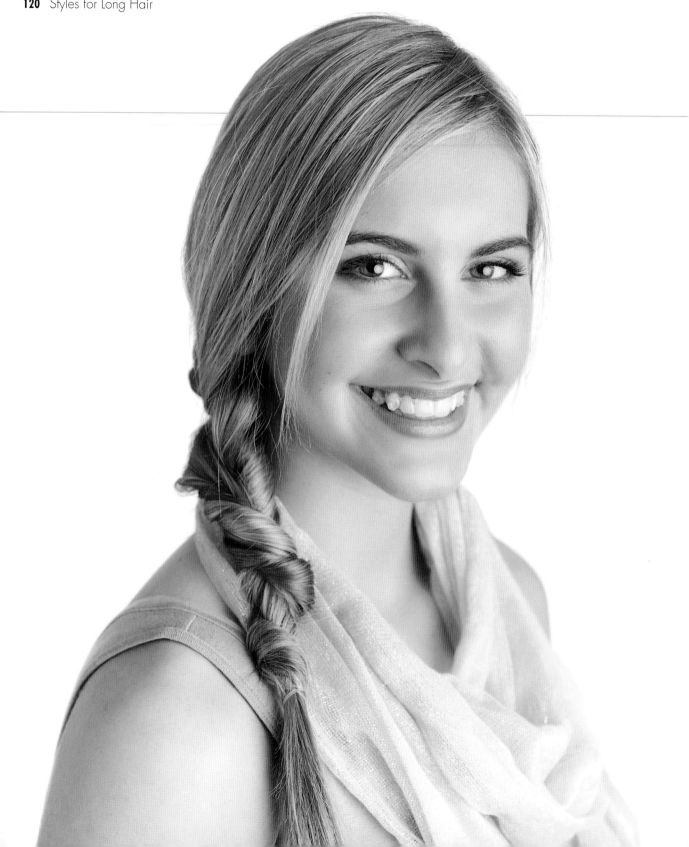

Bear Claw Ponytail

LONG

At first sight, the woven twists of this ponytail bring to mind a bear's claws. And while you could certainly wear this casual look for a hike in the great outdoors, it works just as well for wandering round market stalls, or rocking out at a summer festival. This low-slung side twist can also be transformed into a dressier bun. All hair types can twist into this style.

For a little more volume, apply a few sprays of dry shampoo to your roots and massage in. If you want lots more volume, use a backcombing comb to backcomb the hair at your crown.

TOOLS NEEDED

- hair grips (optional)
- clear hair elastics
- sectioning clips
- hairpins (optional)
- tail comb
- dry shampoo (optional)

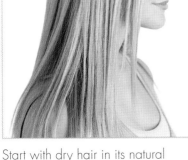

1

Start with dry hair in its natural state, whether straight, wavy, or curly.

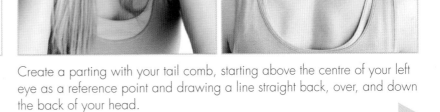

2

Create a parting with your tail comb, starting above the centre of your left eye as a reference point and drawing a line straight back, over, and down the back of your head.

▶

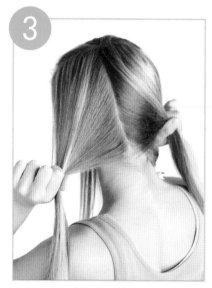

Keeping the left section low at the nape of your neck, separate it into two equal-sized subsections. You can use a clip to keep the other section out of the way.

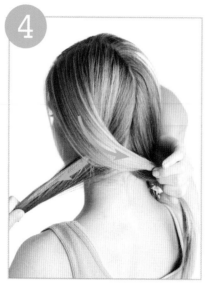

Hold the right subsection down with one hand and, using your other hand, twist the left subsection over the right. Now the right is on the left and the left is on the right.

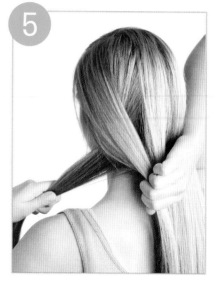

Unclip the hair from the right side. Grab a vertical section of hair parallel to your first section in step 2, and add that section into the right side of your twist.

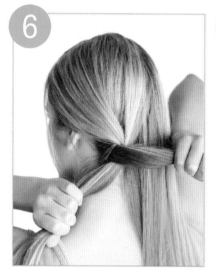

Hold your now thicker right subsection down towards the nape of your neck, as you twist the left side over the right.

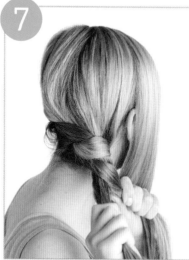

Continue with steps 5 and 6 until your twist reaches the opposite side of your head. Once at that side, add your fringe or your front section of hair into the ponytail. Or leave the fringe out for a more casual look.

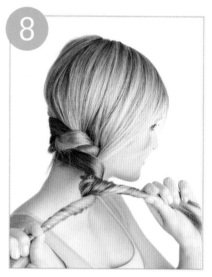

Continue to twist your hair downwards to the very ends of your hair. To keep your twisted pony from unravelling, twist each section in opposite directions. Secure with a clear elastic.

Curly tails

For a variation on this ponytail, stop twisting when you reach the opposite side of your head, secure the twist, and leave the ends of your hair hanging down as a loose ponytail. If you don't have naturally wavy or curly hair, try curling the ponytail with medium-barrel curling tongs. Then take a small piece of hair and wrap it around the ponytail to cover the clear elastic, securing it in place with a hair grip.

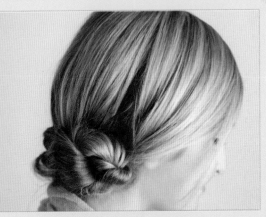

Fancy buns

Once you have secured your twist, you can wrap it up into a bun and fasten it with hairpins for a fancier look.

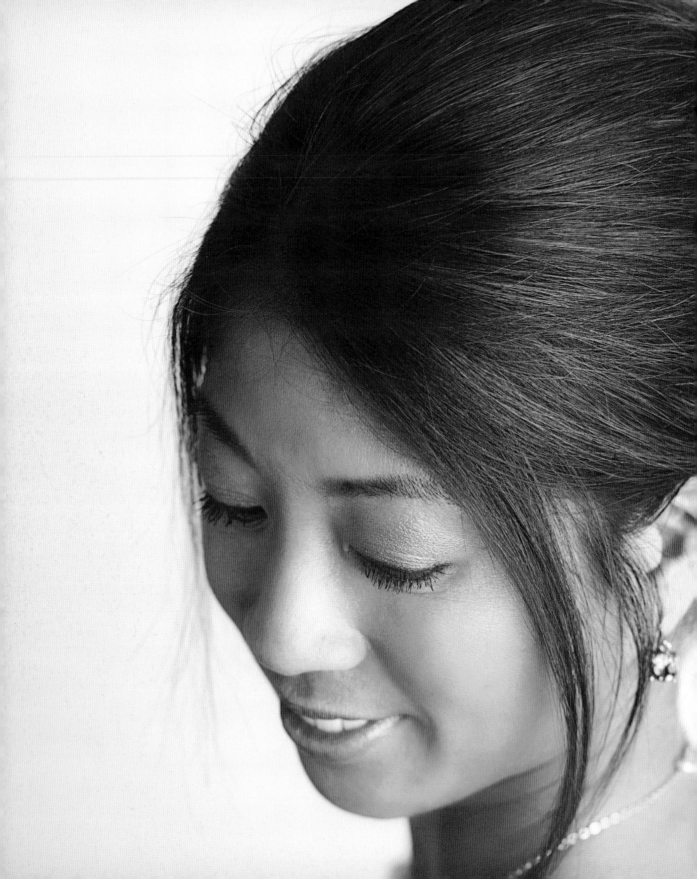

Styles for Special Occasions

When a special occasion arises, what are your first thoughts? What to wear? Which shoes? How you'll style your hair? If this is your line of thinking, you're far from alone. Open a magazine, log on to a website, or turn on the television, and you'll be dazzled by the wonderful hairstyles gracing runway and red carpet alike. Think you can't possibly re-create those styles at home? Think again. In most cases, they're not nearly as tricky as they look.

This section features such classic styles as the Simple Chignon and French Twist, as well as new looks, such as the Broken Fishbone and Side-Swept Pony. With a bit of practice, you'll soon be creating your own polished, professional-looking up-dos and formal styles for parties, weddings, and other special events.

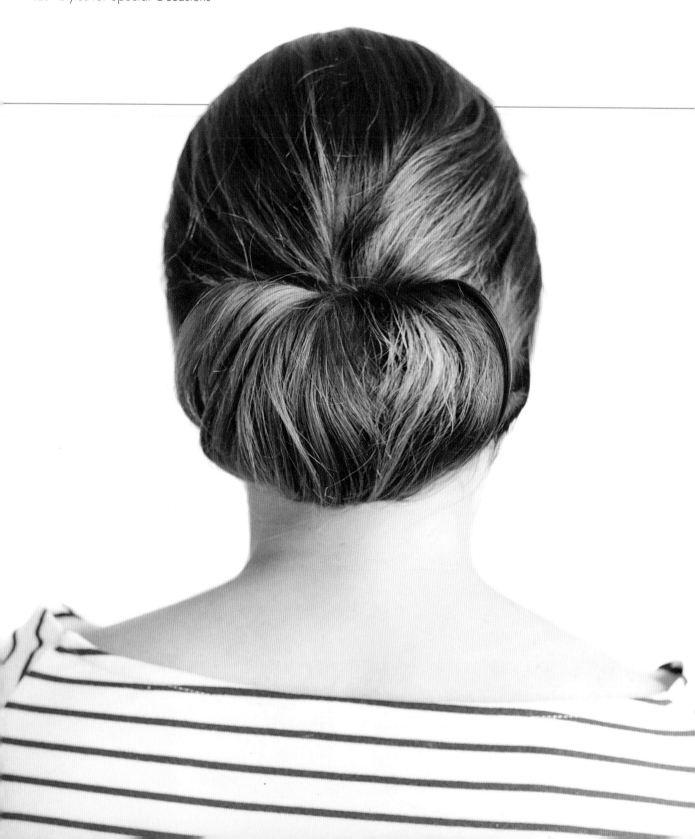

Simple Chignon

OCCASION

When you walk into a room wearing this chic bun, you'll exude elegance. This formal style is a classic type of low-slung bun and it can be a jumping-off point for a variety of other looks. Try a more casual, modern version during the day, wearing it with a headband for a boho twist. The dressier interpretation can take you from a special party to walking down the aisle on your wedding day.

The possibilities with this elegant, timeless style are endless for all hair textures. You can leave your hair in its natural state – straight or curly – to begin this style.

TOOLS NEEDED

- hair grips
- clear hair elastic
- hairpins (optional)
- medium- to firm-hold hairspray
- tail comb
- backcombing comb

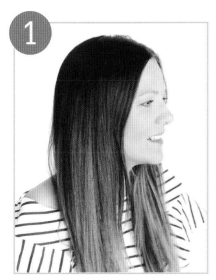

1

Start with dry hair in its natural state, whether it's straight, wavy, or curly.

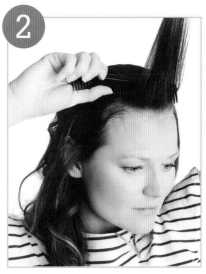

2

Separate off a section of hair about 2.5cm from your hairline. Hold this hair up at 90 degrees from your scalp and gently tease it with the backcombing comb.

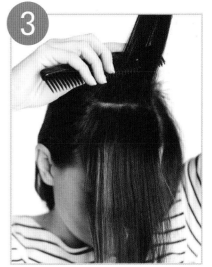

3

Separate a second section in the crown area, directly behind the first, and backcomb that section, too.

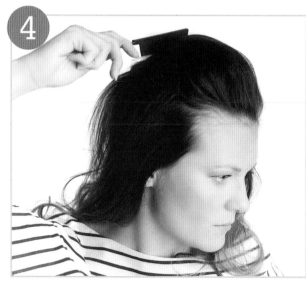

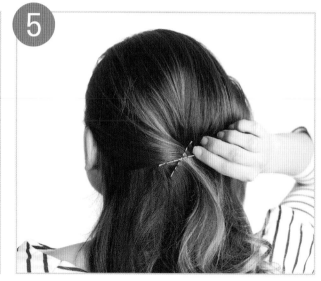

Continue backcombing your hair at the crown until you have lots of volume on top. For additional fullness, backcomb at the sides as well. Use a tail comb to very carefully comb over the backcombed area to smooth the rough edges.

Pick up one side of your hair, as though putting it half-up, and swing it to the back of your head. Secure this section with hair grips, crossing two grips in an X shape to hold it securely.

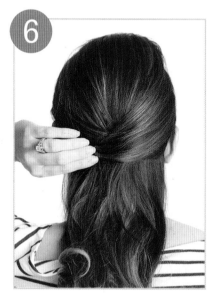

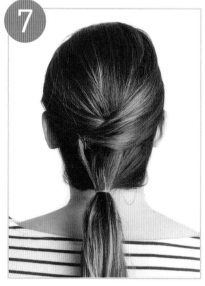

Repeat step 5 with the other side of your hair, pinning this section up and under the first, so the pins don't show. You should now have a voluminous half-up hairdo.

Gather all of your hair, including the bottom of your half-up hairdo, and secure into a loose, low ponytail using a clear elastic.

Keep it casual

For a slightly more casual look, try this with a hairband. After step 7, put a headband around your head about 2.5cm to 5cm from your hairline, or just behind your fringe, placing it over and on top of the elastic. When you make an opening for the ponytail to slip through, do this above the band, so you can pull the hair around the headband as you invert the ponytail.

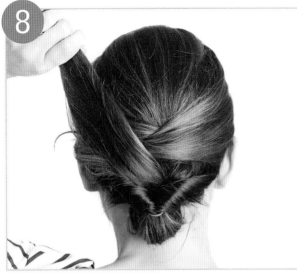

Create a small opening above the elastic at the base of the ponytail, using two fingers. Reach down through the opening, grab the ponytail, and pull it up through the opening.

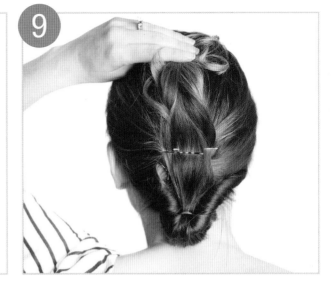

Repeat step 8 to invert your ponytail again, and pin it horizontally with hair grips.

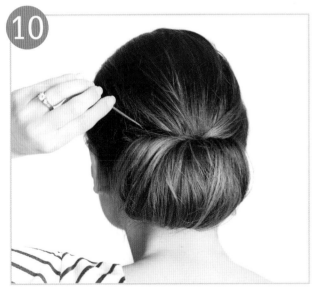

Tuck the remaining ends of your ponytail down at the nape of your neck to produce a bun. Secure any loose ends with hairpins and/or hair grips. Finish with a medium- to firm-hold hairspray to tame any unruly strands and set the style.

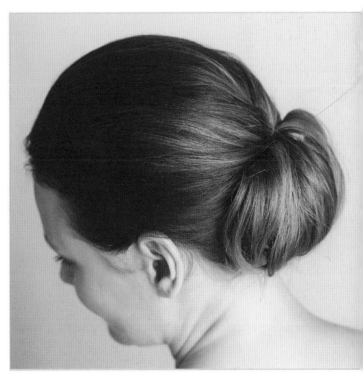

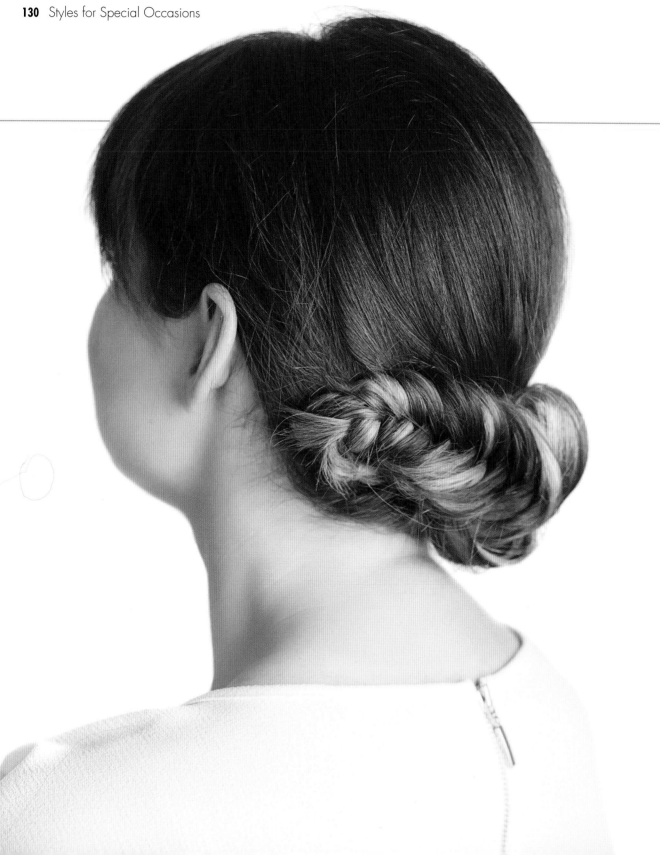

Fishtail Bun

The Fishtail Bun is an earthy, unpretentious style that's eye-catching nonetheless. If you're a fan of the messy bun, you'll love this look. It's a simple and low-maintenance hairdo with high-maintenance appeal. This low-slung bun works as a casual weekend look, but it could just as easily be worn when walking down the aisle. All hair except extremely curly types (it's better to blow-dry curly hair straighter first) can achieve this style – and it only takes about 10 minutes.

Before blow-drying, use a holding product to help your style last longer. You don't want pieces of your hair to come undone. Use a volumizer on your roots for lift at the crown, and either a volumizing foam or sculpting lotion for the middle and ends of your hair.

TOOLS NEEDED

- antihumidity hairspray
- hairdryer with concentrator nozzle
- volumizing foam or sculpting lotion
- hair grips
- clear hair elastics
- hairpins
- paddle brush
- backcombing comb (optional)

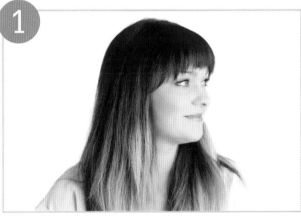

Start with thoroughly towel-dried hair.

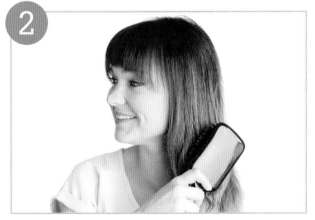

Apply a holding product evenly throughout your hair, and use a paddle brush to further distribute the product by brushing until smooth.

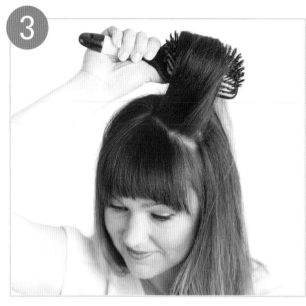

Using the paddle brush, pick up a section of hair at the roots and slightly turn the brush up and back to create a little bubble in your hair.

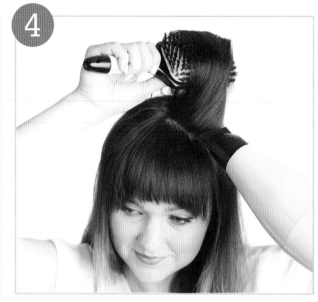

Point the hairdryer, fitted with a concentrator nozzle, close to the roots and up towards the brush holding the bubbled-over hair. This creates volume without the need to round brush or backcomb your whole head.

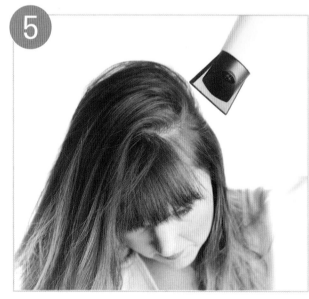

Continue drying the rest of your hair in a back and forth motion until it's dry.

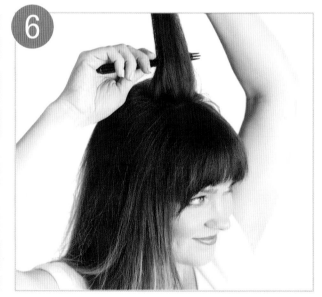

When your hair is completely dry, you can, if you like, use a backcombing comb to backcomb the crown area for more volume.

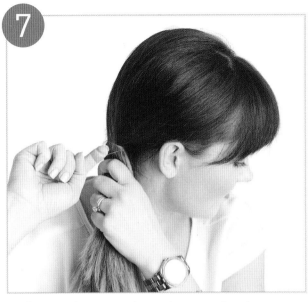

Gather your hair into a low side ponytail and secure it with a clear elastic.

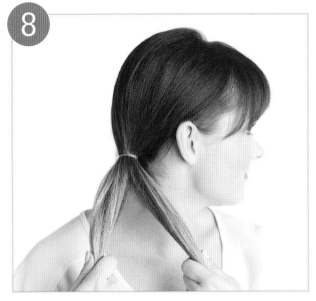

Divide your ponytail into two equal sections.

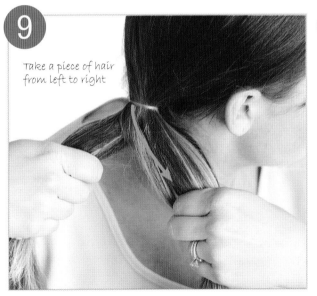

Take a piece of hair from left to right

Pick up a piece of hair from the far left side of the left section, and cross it over the top and into the right section. This piece is now a part of the right section.

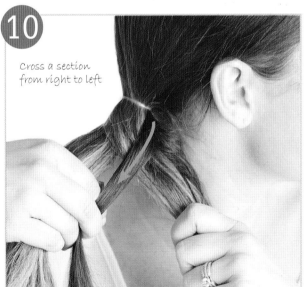

Cross a section from right to left

Pick up a piece of hair on the outer right side of the right section, and pull it over and into the left section. That small section is now a part of the left side.

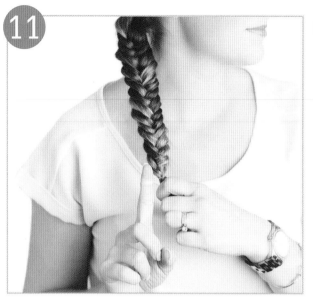

Repeat steps 9 and 10 until your entire ponytail is fishtail plaited. Secure the ends with a clear hair elastic.

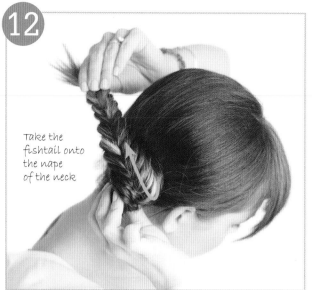

Take the fishtail onto the nape of the neck

Flip the fishtail upwards, onto the hair at the nape of your neck. The fishtail is now flipped up and to the opposite side.

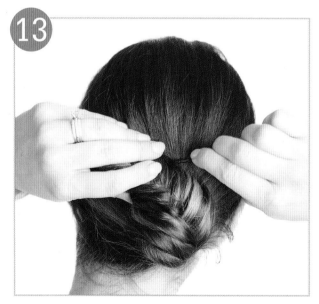

Secure the fishtail with hairpins, pinning the sides of the tail into the hair at the base of your original ponytail.

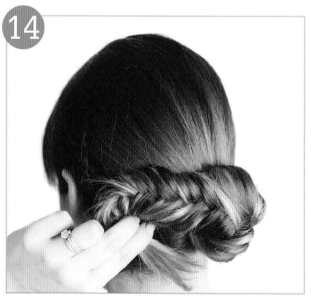

When the fishtail is secure against your head, tuck under the ends and secure with a hair grip. Try to hide the clear elastic if you can.

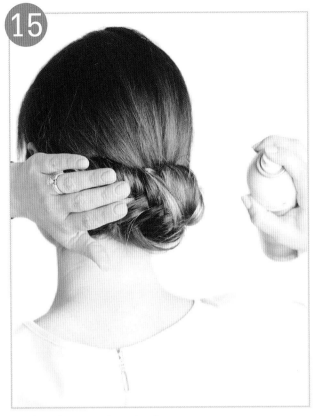

Finish with an antihumidity hairspray.

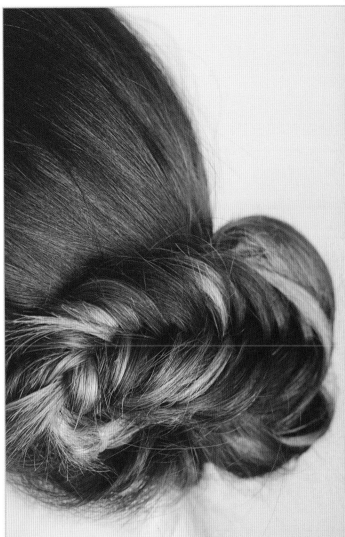

Dreamy look

For an ethereal feel, you can pull the fishtail apart a little to make it looser and slightly messy. Pin any additional unruly hairs with hairpins.

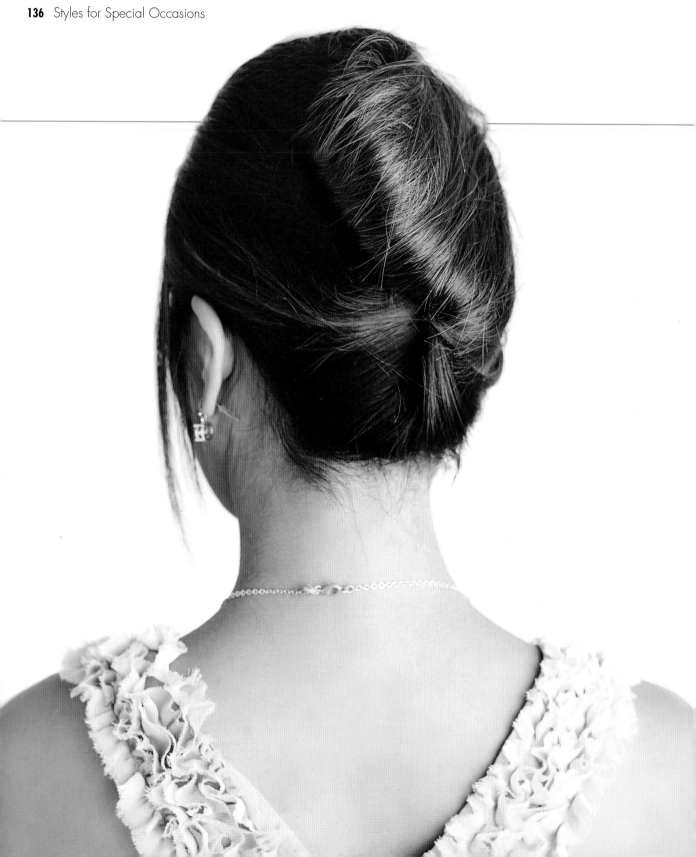

French Twist

OCCASION

The French Twist was the height of fashion in the 1960s and has remained a classic style ever since. This up-do is très chic and is often worn at formal parties, weddings, and even in office settings. More recently, the French Twist has transformed into a more casual style with a loose and airy feel, perfect for those with more natural texture in their hair.

TOOLS NEEDED

- sectioning clips (optional)
- hairpins
- hairspray
- paddle brush
- backcombing comb

You want your hair to be relatively smooth to start this style. If you have curly or wavy locks, blow-dry them straighter first. If you have straight hair, this step might not be necessary, but it can help give the finished style extra smoothness.

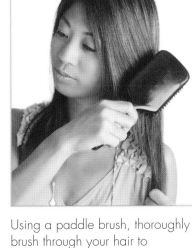

1 Start with dry hair.

2 Using a paddle brush, thoroughly brush through your hair to remove any tangles or snags and promote smoothness.

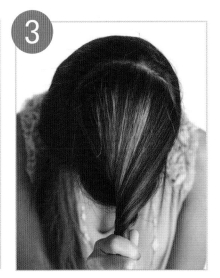

3 Part out a small section of hair from the corner of your hairline on one side to the other in a U shape. You can clip the bottom section out of the way. ▶

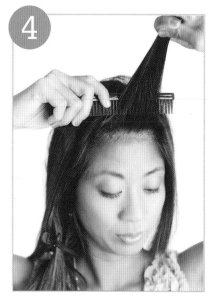

Using the comb, backcomb this entire section to create soft, subtle volume.

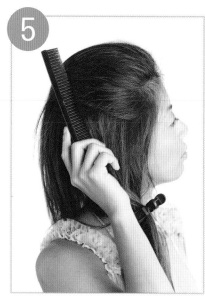

After you've finished backcombing, very gently comb the outer layer to smooth it.

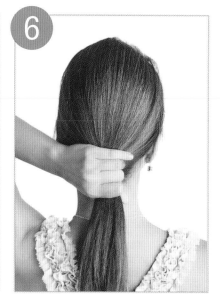

Gather your hair into a low, central ponytail.

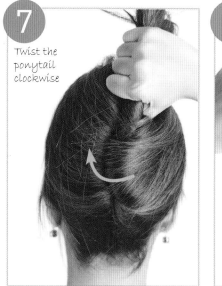

Twist the ponytail clockwise

Twist your ponytail clockwise, moving your hand slightly upwards until the twist is upside down, with the ends of your hair reaching up past your crown.

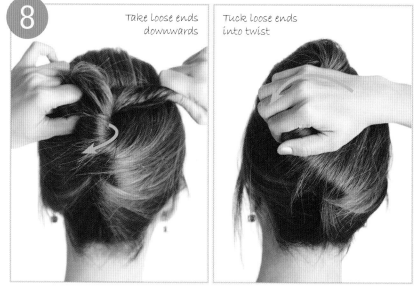

Take loose ends downwards

Tuck loose ends into twist

Fold the loose ends of hair downwards and tuck them into the twist. You can use your other hand to help fold over the twisted section.

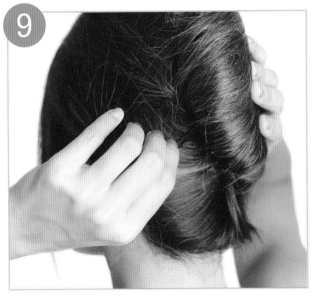

After you've tucked as much as possible into the twist, secure all the loose ends with hairpins.

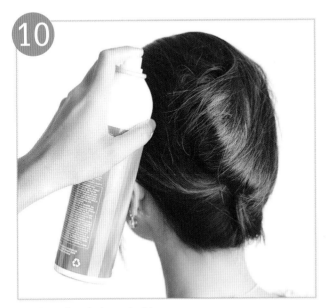

Finish with a light veil of hairspray.

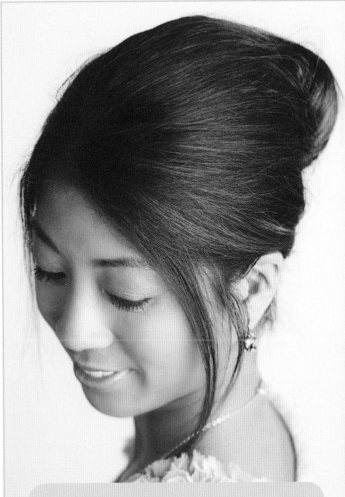

Enhancing the look

You can skip the pins and use a decorative comb instead. Many brides have used this accessory to add a little sparkle to their wedding-day style. If you opt for this look, spray your comb with hairspray first, and tame any flyaways with an antihumidity pomade. You can use some shine spray to give your hair extra gloss, too.

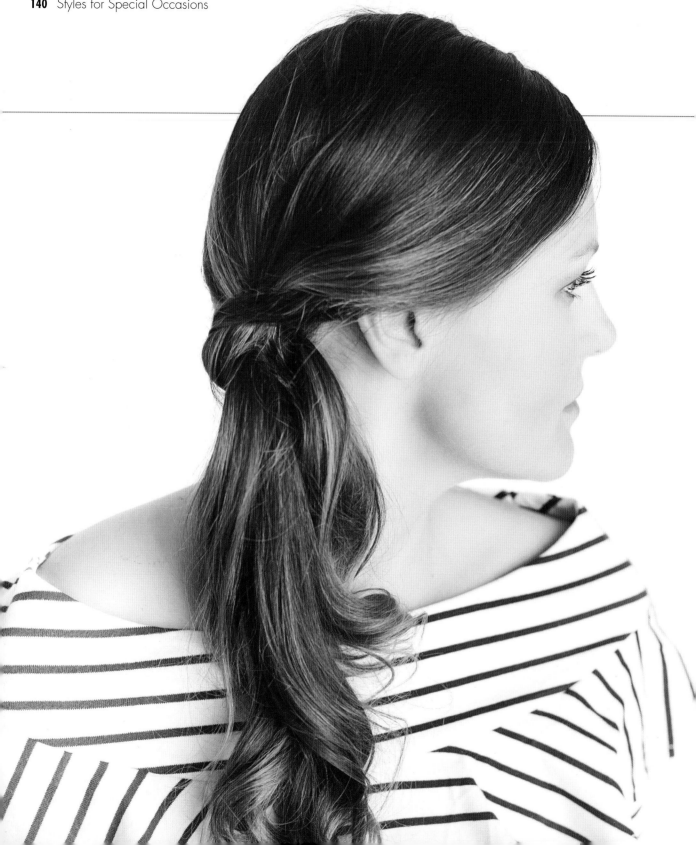

Side-Swept Pony

The Side-Swept Pony, an unpretentious special-occasion style, has become hugely popular, especially with teens dressing up for the prom, bridesmaids, and even brides. And thanks to American music stars like Taylor Swift, this ponytail doesn't seem to be going out of style any time soon. All hair types can achieve this look.

TOOLS NEEDED

- hair grips
- clear hair elastics
- sectioning clips
- curling tongs with a 2.5cm or 3cm barrel
- curl clips
- hairpins (optional)
- backcombing comb

For this look, you want to start with plenty of natural volume. You can blow-dry your hair straighter if you have wavy or curly locks, but make sure that you still keep some volume.

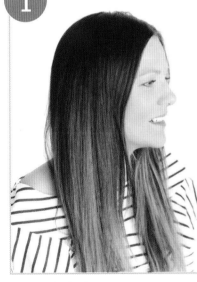

Start with dry hair.

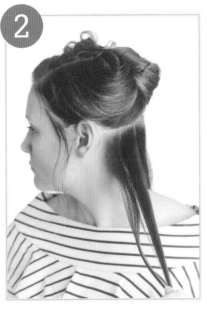

Using 2.5cm or 3cm curling tongs, and working with 5cm sections for more efficient curls, curl your hair away from your face.

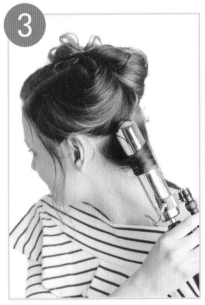

Curl each strand from the root to the tip for a more voluminous look.

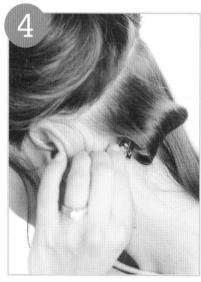

As you finish each curl, drop the curl lightly into your palm, wrap the curl back up around your fingers, place a curl clip inside the curl, and clip it to the hair at your scalp to set the curl.

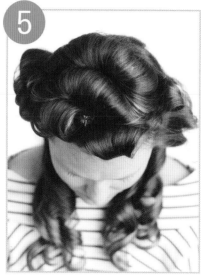

Continue curling and pinning until your entire head is full of pinned curls. After your curls have cooled completely (5 to 10 minutes), remove the clips.

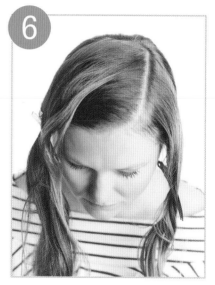

Separate your hair into two sections, front and back, by parting from the top of one ear to the other. Clip all the hair in the front along your hairline out of the way.

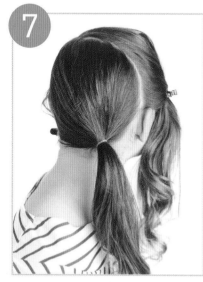

Gather the back section of your hair into a low side ponytail, so that it rests on your shoulder, and secure it with a clear hair elastic.

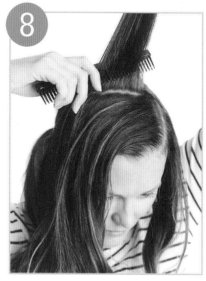

Release the front section. Using a backcombing comb, backcomb the crown and then gently comb over it to smooth out any unruly bits.

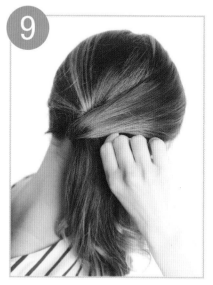

Wrap that top section over your low side ponytail. Using hair grips or hairpins, pin to secure the top section to the bottom.

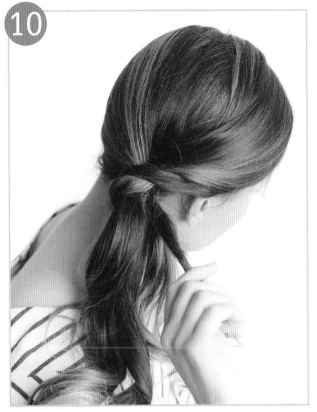

10

Take the final section of hair from the front on the side of your parting, and either twist this section in front of your ponytail to hide the elastic, or wrap it around the elastic. Secure it with a hair grip, leaving the ends down to mingle with your ponytail.

Additional touches

Depending on the length of your fringe or your layers at the front, you can pull a few pieces of hair loose to soften the look. And for extra sparkle, add a decorative barrette or slide to your ponytail.

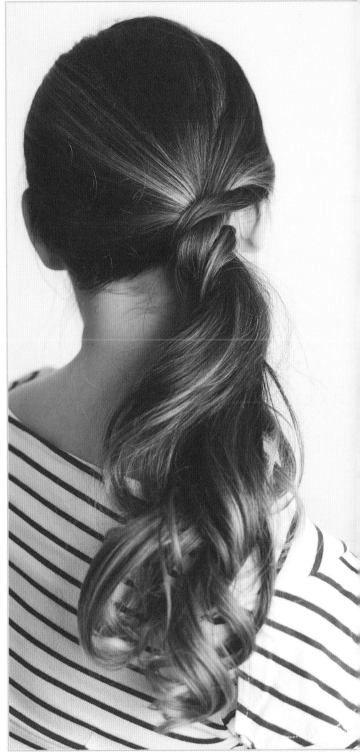

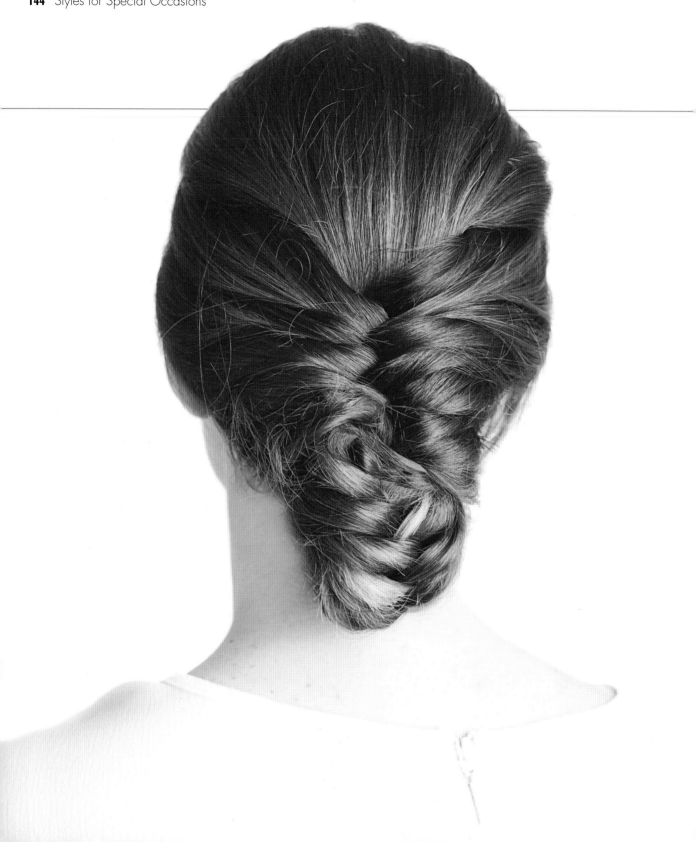

Broken Fishbone

OCCASION

This modern up-do will earn you lots of attention – your friends will beg you to tell them how you did it. The Broken Fishbone is a chignon that appears to be especially intricate but is actually quite simple. Brides look radiant with this style, and it's great for anyone looking for a fresh new twist on evening-out hair. All hair textures can achieve this look.

Before starting this style, if your hair is naturally straight, use curling tongs with a 5cm barrel to add some texture.

TOOLS NEEDED

- hair grips
- clear hair elastics
- hairpins (optional)
- tail comb

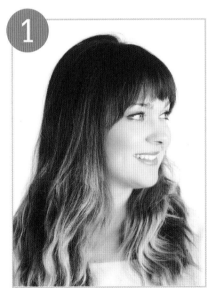

Start with dry hair.

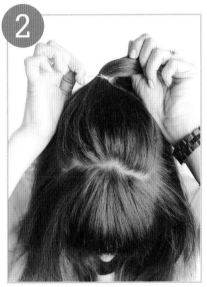

Using a tail comb, gather a U-shaped section of hair at the crown, from one corner of your hairline to the other. Secure this section of hair at the back of your head with a clear elastic.

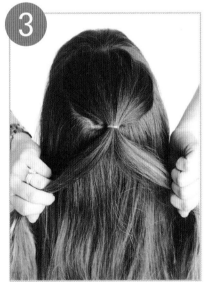

Divide the small ponytail into two equal sections.

▶

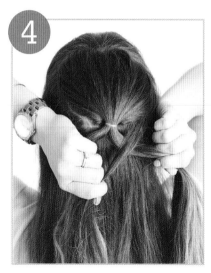

Pick up a horizontal section of hair directly beneath the ponytail on the right side. Cross this section of hair over and add it to the left section your left hand is holding.

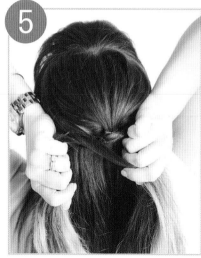

Pick up a horizontal section beneath the ponytail area on the left side. Cross it over and add it to the right section. Your right hand remains holding the right section.

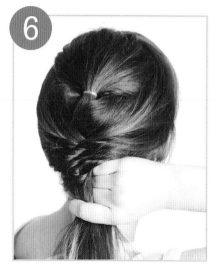

Repeat steps 4 and 5 until you reach the nape of your neck.

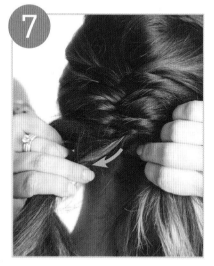

When you reach your nape, begin to plait the rest of your hair in a classic fishtail, grabbing a small outer piece of hair from the right side and crossing it over and into the left section.

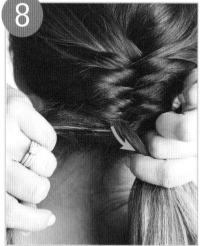

Next, grab a small outer section of hair from the left side and cross it over and into the right side. Keep your right hand on the right section of hair and your left hand on the left section the whole time.

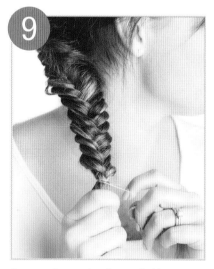

Secure the ends of your fishbone plait with another clear elastic.

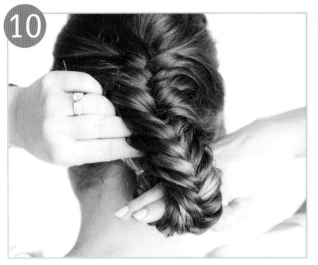

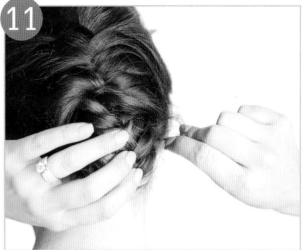

Wrap the end of the fishbone tail around your index and middle fingers to coil it upwards.

Curl the coil up to the French-plaited fishtail, tuck it up and underneath, and secure it with hair grips. You can add hairpins for any layers or stray hairs that have fallen out of place during the styling process.

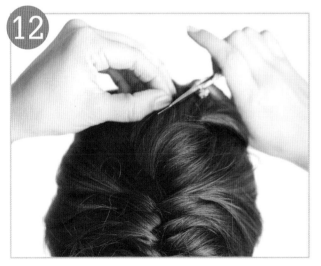

If your fishtail is low and doesn't cover the first elastic, you can cut and remove this elastic.

Boho chic

For added glamour and urban hippie appeal, add a headscarf or headband.

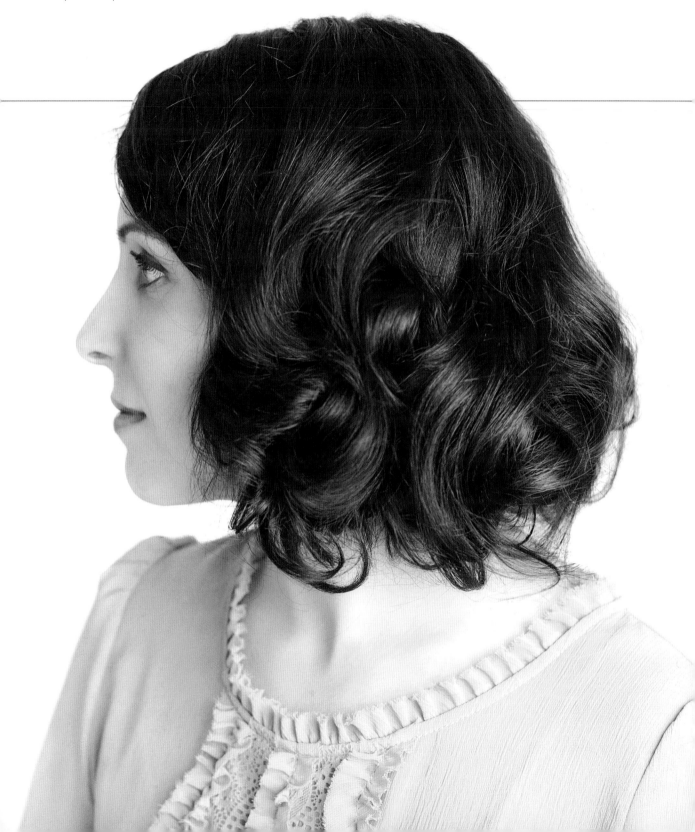

Faux Bob

OCCASION

Love your longer hair but sometimes yearn for a short-hair look? This style allows you to have short hair temporarily, without actually getting the chop. The Faux Bob has a vintage glam allure that suits special events – it makes frequent appearances on the red carpet.

Though this look is best for dressier occasions, it can be transformed into a more casual style with a couple of tweaks.

TOOLS NEEDED

- boar bristle brush
- hair grips
- clear hair elastics
- sectioning clips
- curling tongs with a 2.5cm barrel
- curl clips
- firm-hold hairspray
- hairpins (optional)
- backcombing comb

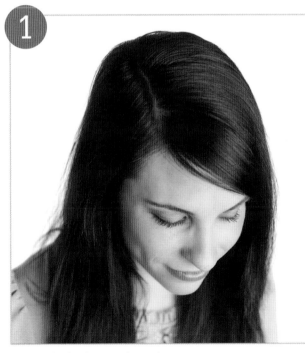

Start with dry hair and a side parting.

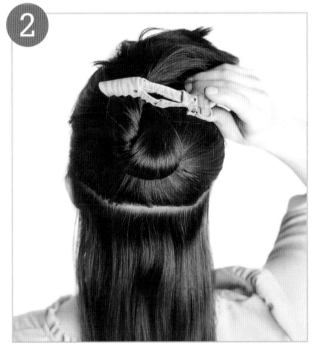

Part your hair horizontally from the top of one ear, around the back of your head, to the top of the other ear. Clip the top section of hair up and out of the way. ▶

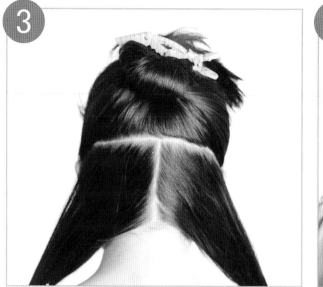

Divide the bottom section into two equal sections.

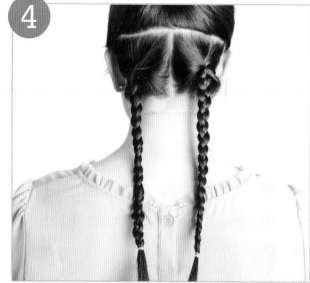

Plait both sections and secure the ends of the plaits with clear elastics.

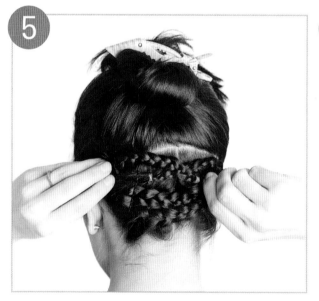

Fold the plaits up onto the bottom of the back of your head, so they lie as flat as possible. You want them up out of the way against your scalp, so they will be hidden underneath the top section of your hair later. Secure the plaits in place with hair grips.

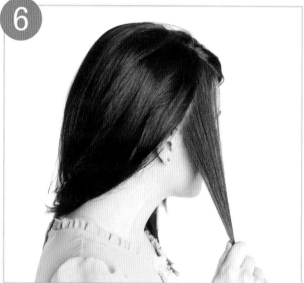

Release the top section of hair and divide it into small vertical subsections to prepare for curling.

7

Curl towards
your face

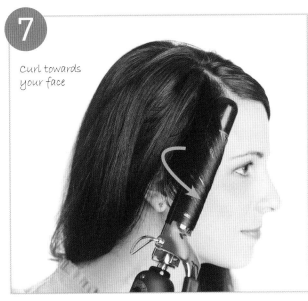

Using 2.5cm curling tongs, curl each subsection forwards, towards your face.

8

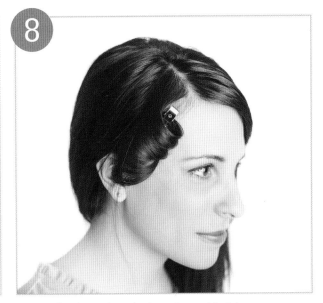

As you finish each curl, drop the curl lightly into your palm, wrap the curl back up around your fingers, place a curl clip inside the curl, and clip it to the hair at your scalp to set.

9

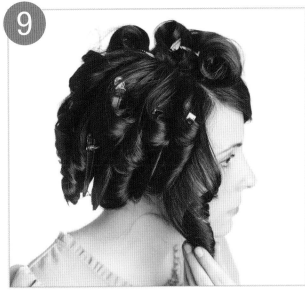

After your entire head has been curled and set with the curl clips, remove each clip very carefully, so you don't disrupt the curls.

10

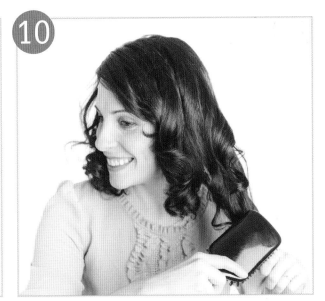

Thoroughly brush through your hair with a boar bristle brush to soften the curls.

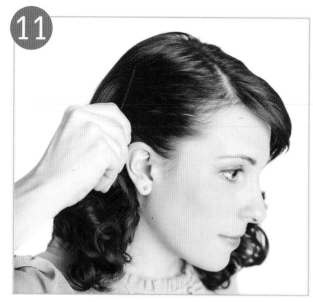

Use a hair grip to pin one side of your hair back behind your ear, on the same side as your parting.

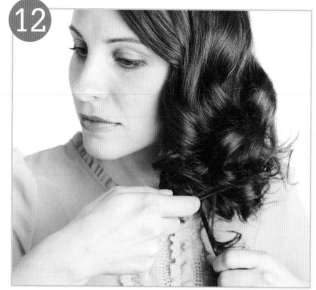

Using a backcombing comb, backcomb the ends of your hair to give them added fullness.

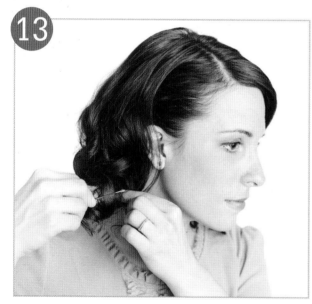

Begin pinning the ends of your hair by tucking the sections up and under and securing with hair grips or hairpins. Pin just above the ends of your hair, so the ends can hang down and make your bob look more realistic. The pins will have plenty to grip onto, as you pin into the plaits hidden underneath your bob.

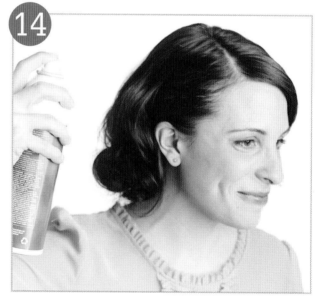

Finish with a firm-hold hairspray. If you're likely to be dancing later, you don't want this style to come undone.

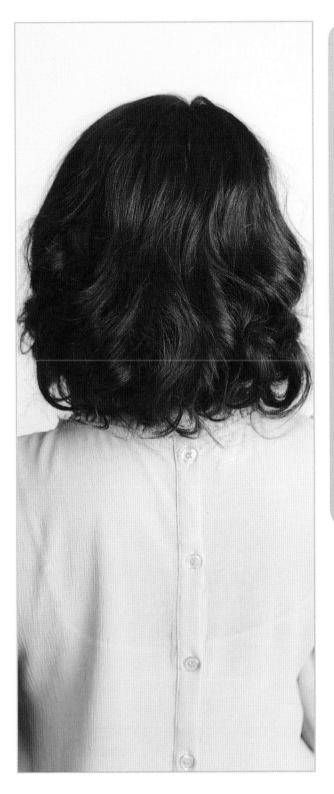

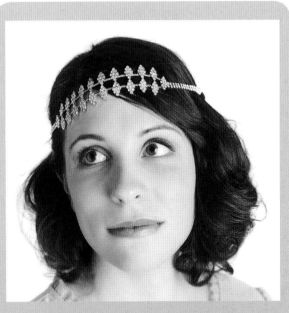

Modifying the bob

After all your hair has been pinned up, slip a headband over the top for the vintage flapper look.

For a more casual style, forgo the headband, and pull out a couple of pieces of hair at your hairline. This creates a softer, slightly undone look.

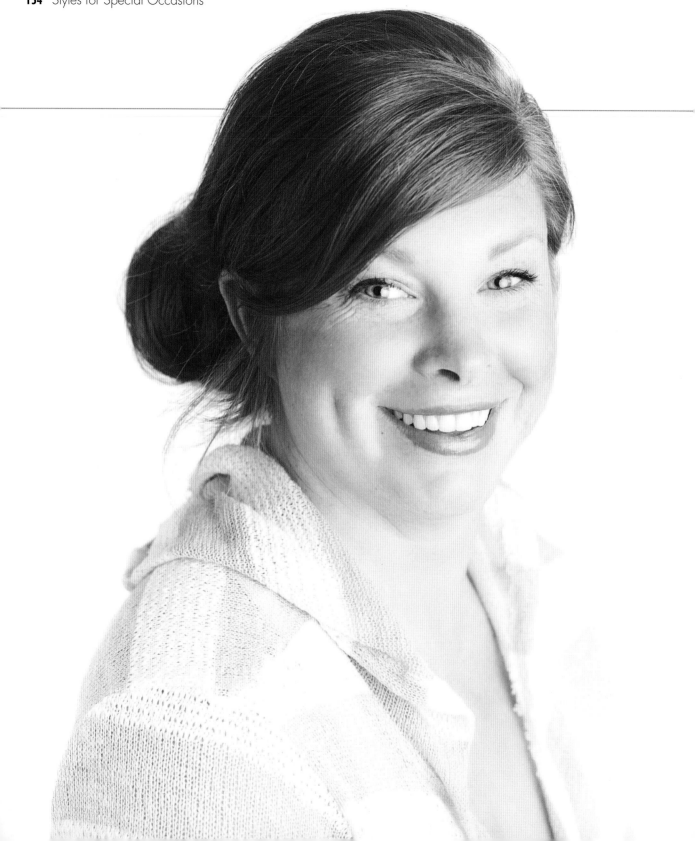

Side Bun

A variation on the classic bun, the Side Bun will quickly become an essential part of your hairstyle repertoire. This look is particularly good for weddings, or any special gathering that calls for a refined, elegant style. All hair types can achieve this style, which appears far more time-consuming than it really is.

You don't need to do much preparation for this style. If you have extremely curly hair, you might want to blow-dry it to loosen your curls. Whatever texture hair you have, you want to eliminate frizz as much as possible.

TOOLS NEEDED

- hair grips
- clear hair elastics
- sectioning clips
- curling tongs with a 3cm to 5cm barrel
- hairpins (optional)
- long sectioning clips
- medium- to firm-hold hairspray
- backcombing comb

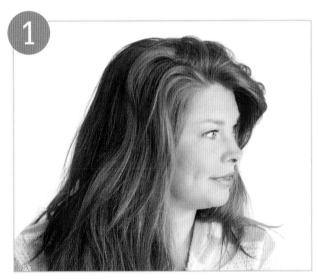

Start with dry hair.

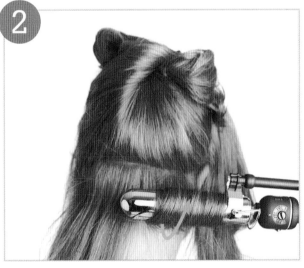

Part your hair horizontally from the top of one ear, behind your head, to the top of your other ear, and clip the top section out of the way. Separate your hair into small subsections and use 3cm to 5cm curling tongs to curl your hair upwards.

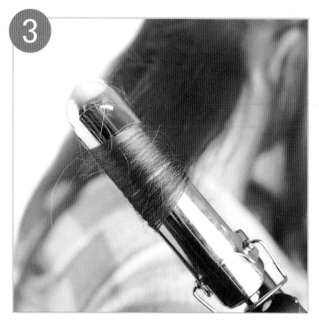

Be sure to include the very tip of each strand in the curl. This ensures the curl is as smooth as possible.

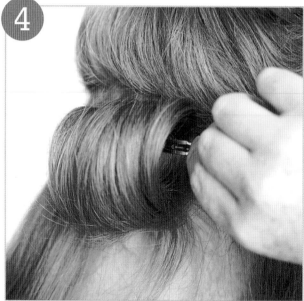

Release the curl from the barrel, roll it back up into the curled position, and secure it to your head with a long sectioning clip.

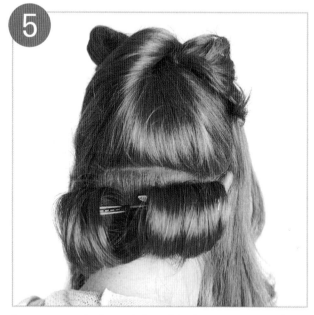

Repeat steps 2, 3, and 4 until the bottom section of your hair is all curled and clipped. After all your curls are set and cool (5 to 10 minutes), remove the clips.

Avoiding creases

Be sure to use flat sectioning clips instead of regular curl clips. These will allow your hair to set without leaving any creases.

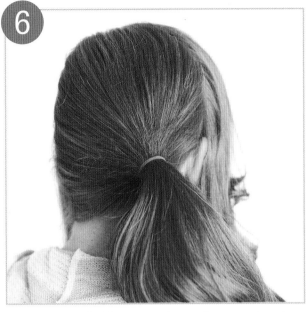

Gather your curled hair into a low side ponytail and secure it with a clear elastic.

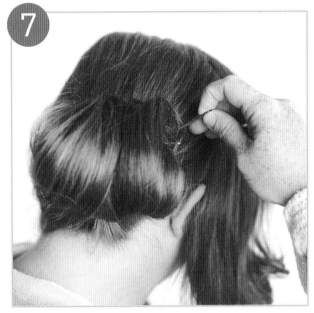

Your hair should naturally want to curl upwards in the ponytail. Roll the ponytail upwards, and secure it with hair grips to the base of your scalp.

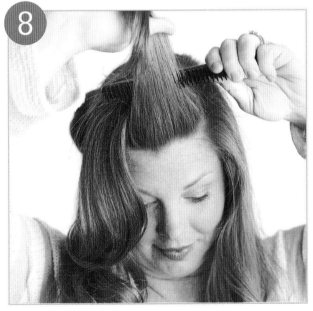

Release the top section of hair and backcomb the crown at the roots to create volume.

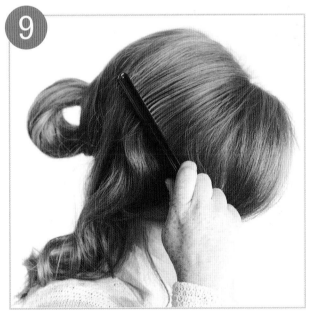

Gently comb over the backcombed section to smooth out any rough patches.

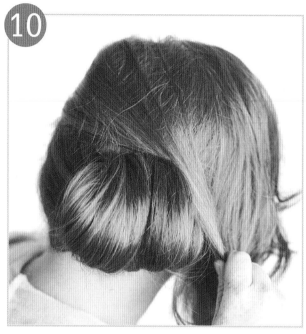

Wrap the ends of the top section around the low bun, and pin any loose hair up and underneath the bun with hairpins or hair grips.

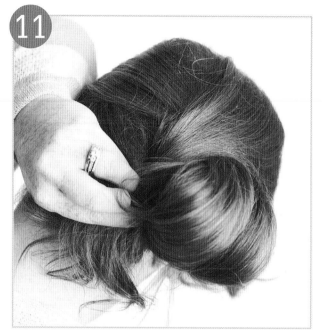

Pull the left side of the bun over to the right side.

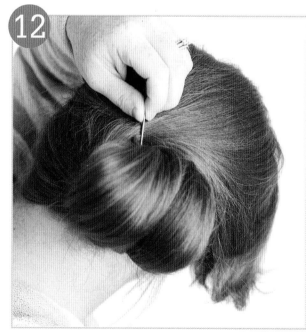

Pin this piece in place with hair grips or hairpins.

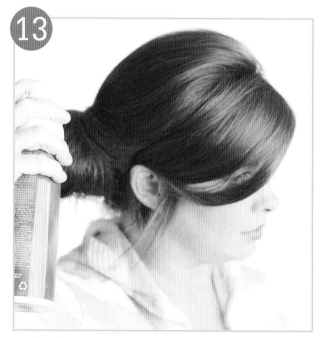

Finish with a medium- to firm-hold hairspray.

Adding softness

If you want to soften up this style, you can pull out your fringe or a few short (not long) front pieces. This gives the style a more relaxed look.

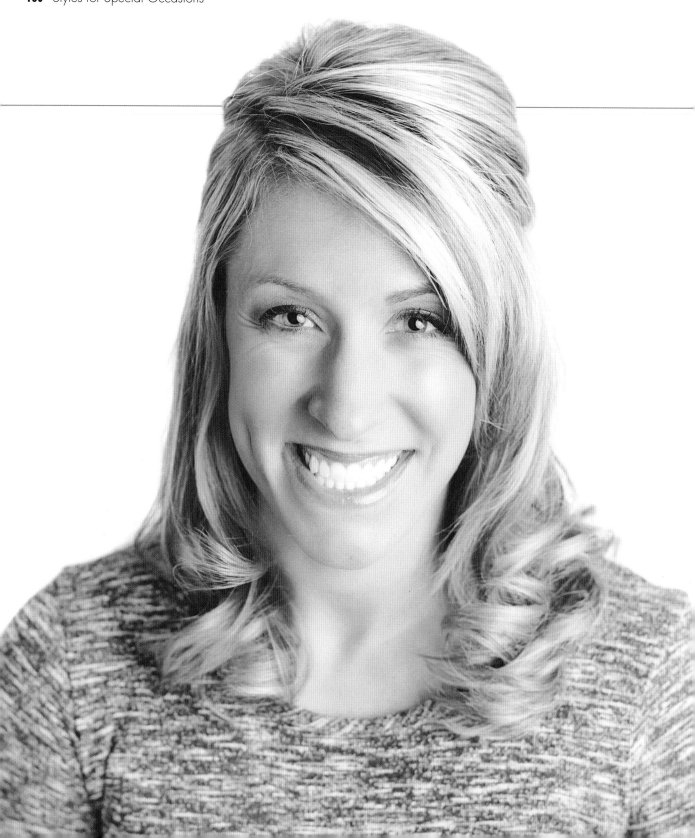

Half Up

OCCASION

Brides around the world are opting for a simpler style for their big day. The Half Up gives a more laid-back feel to the styles typically worn at weddings. It can also be paired with wreaths of flowers for a gorgeous organic halo effect. Although it's more relaxed than a traditional up-do, it still has plenty of polish for that special event. All textures and types of hair can achieve this look.

For a little more volume and grip at the crown, use a root-lifting foam. Apply this directly to your scalp and massage it into the roots of your hair with your fingertips.

TOOLS NEEDED

- hair grips
- curling tongs with a 2.5cm to 3cm barrel
- light-hold hairspray (optional)
- spray wax (optional)
- backcombing comb

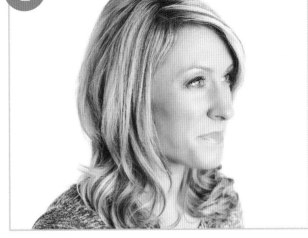

1

For added movement, start with hair that has been allowed to dry naturally.

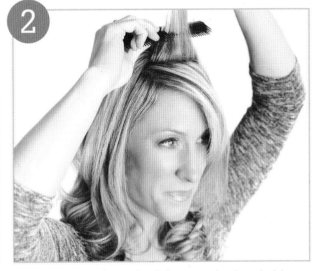

2

Beginning around 5cm back from your hairline, hold a section of hair at 90 degrees to your scalp, and backcomb at the crown. Continue until your entire crown is full of volume.

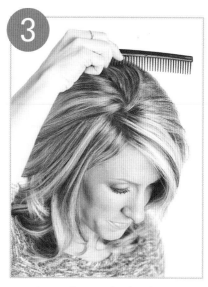

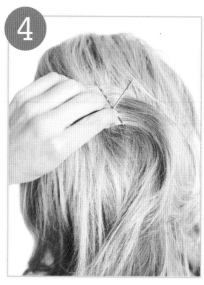

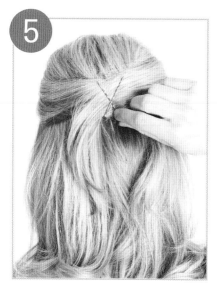

Gently comb over the backcombed area to smooth it, without disrupting all the volume you just created.

Grab a small section of hair just above your left ear, and secure it across the back of your head with two hair grips, crossing them in an X shape.

Grab a small section of hair above your right ear and pull it across the back of your head, past and over the section you just pinned. Pin this section with the X method, too.

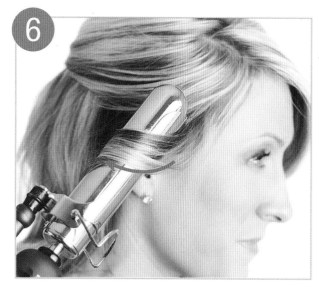

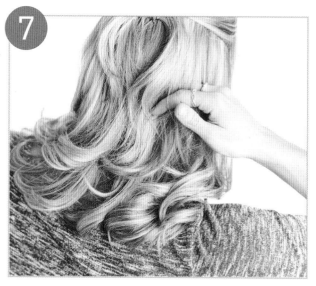

Curl the remainder of your hair hanging down. It's easiest to grab small vertical subsections and curl away from your face, using tongs with a 2.5cm to 3cm barrel.

Using your fingers, gently comb through your curls.

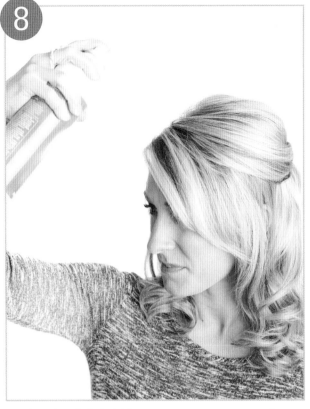

8

Finish with a light-hold hairspray, or a spray wax for additional texture.

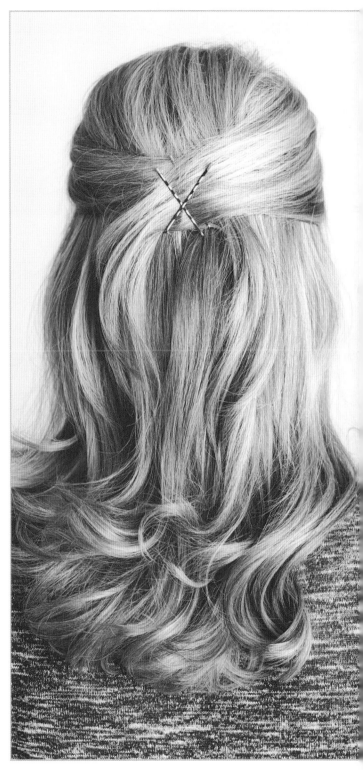

Final touches

For the ultimate romantic look, add a flower garland or a pretty headwrap.

Alternatively, use a decorative flower or bow clip to cover and disguise the hair grips.

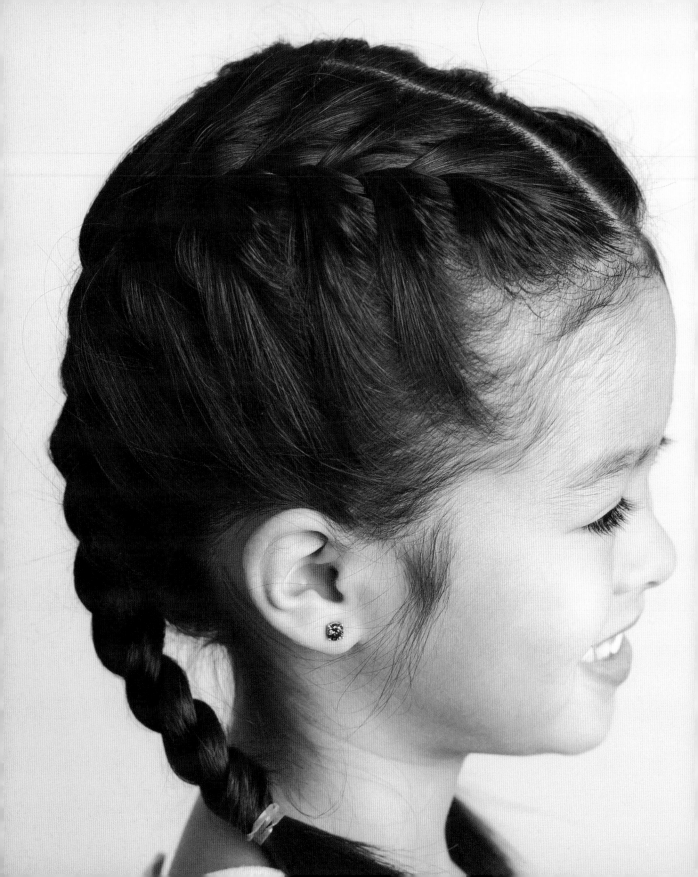

Super Styles
for Girls

It's not only grown-ups who want to ring the changes with their hair. Whether she's your daughter, niece, cousin, or sister, girls of all ages will enjoy wearing the fun and fresh hairstyles covered in this section. Once you've mastered the classic French plait, you'll be able to style her hair in the pretty but practical Double French Plait. Two brand-new styles, the Twisted Sister and Hair Bow, can be dressed up or down to suit occasions ranging from the school prom to family dinners, parties to concert performances. Wherever they're worn, they're bound to make a statement.

Of course, these styles aren't restricted to the younger generation, either – feel free to try them on your own hair, too.

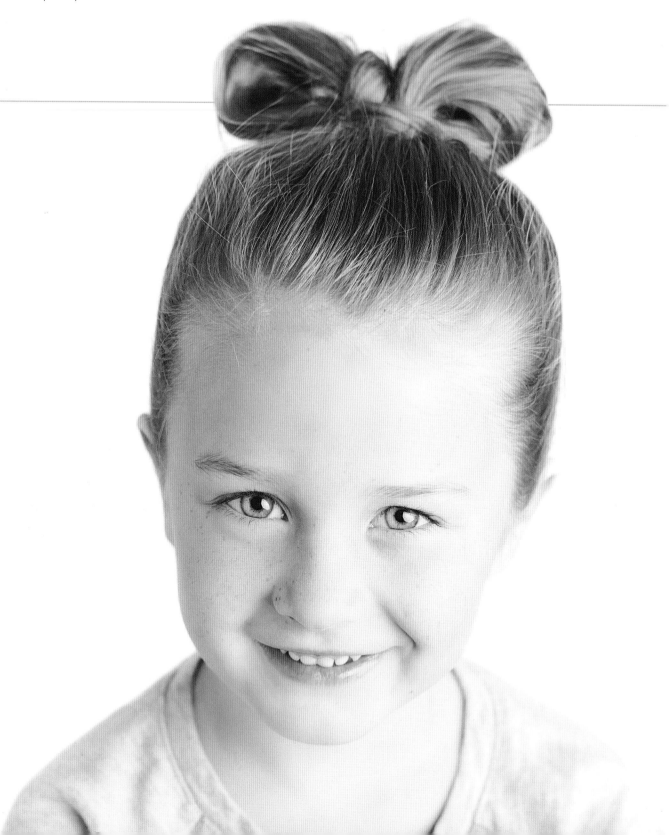

Hair Bow

Bows are always popular with little girls – from examples small enough to fit on a barrette, to bows decorating a ponytail, or oversized bows adorning an Alice band. This hairstyle involves styling her hair into an actual hair bow. It is a great look for a school concert, a family party, or any other special occasion. This style works well with both wavy tresses and straight hair.

If there are flyaways, you can use a bit of defining paste to smooth the hair after backcombing in step 2. If you like, you can also smooth the ponytail with a defining paste before step 4. This helps a layered haircut hold together in the hair bow.

TOOLS NEEDED

- hair grips
- colourful or clear hair elastics
- light-hold hairspray
- backcombing comb
- defining paste (optional)

1

Start with dry hair.

2

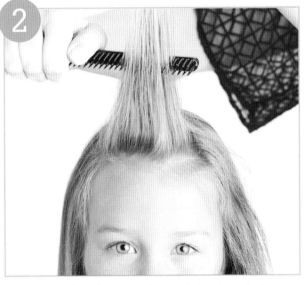

Using a backcombing comb, gently backcomb the crown area slightly for a little extra volume on top. ▶

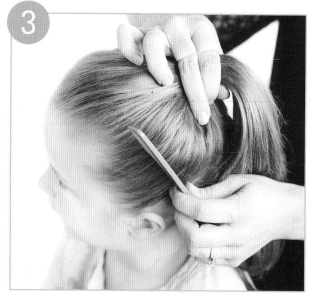

Gather her hair into a high ponytail, using a comb to smooth out any bumps along the way, and secure with a colourful elastic.

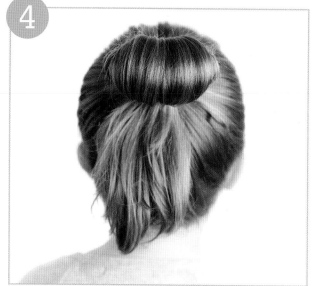

Wrap another elastic around the ponytail, but don't pull the tail all the way through on the last pull. This creates a bun-looking top half, with the ends of the ponytail hanging down at the bottom.

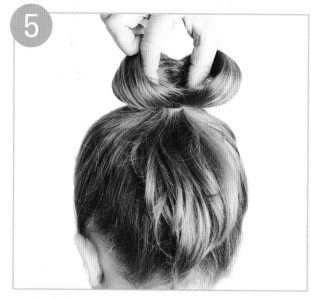

Divide the bun into two down the centre, creating two separate buns.

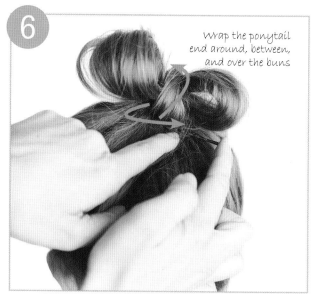

Wrap the ponytail end around, between, and over the buns

Grab a piece of hair from the ends of the ponytail still hanging down and wrap this piece of hair up, around, between, and over the buns. Secure it with a hair grip.

7

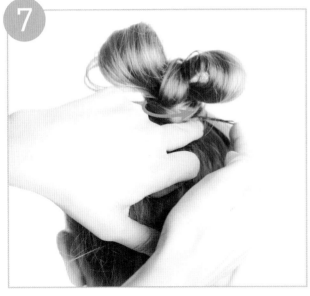

Wrap the remaining piece of hair (from the ends of the ponytail) around the base of the ponytail and secure it with a hair grip.

8

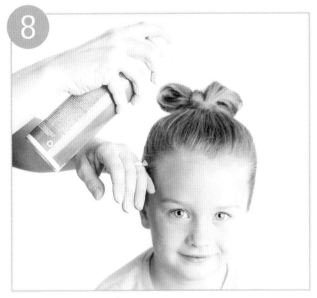

Finish with a light-hold hairspray.

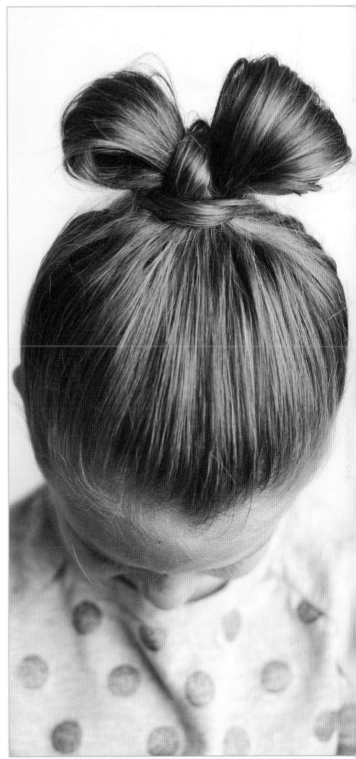

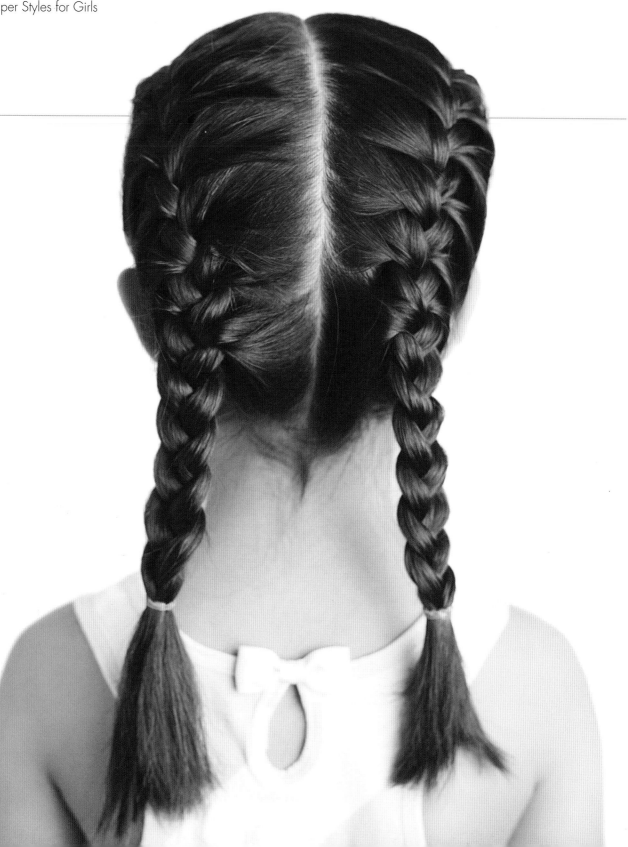

Double French Plait

The French plait is a lovely style on its own, but it's also easy to adapt into different looks. The Double French Plait is simply two French plaits divided by a centre parting. It's a great way to keep the hair out of her face for a sports day or any other activity. All hair textures work well with these plaits.

TOOLS NEEDED

- colourful hair elastics
- hair gel or definining paste
- sectioning clips
- hairspray
- tail comb

If you begin with wet hair, use a medium- to firm-hold hair gel to keep all the little hairs in place. If you start with dry hair, dispense a dollop of defining paste about 2cm in diameter in your palms and distribute it through the lengths of the hair for better grip while you're plaiting.

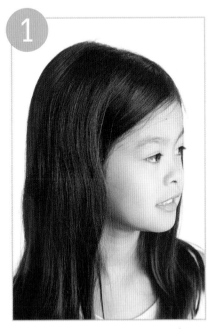

Start with either wet or dry hair.

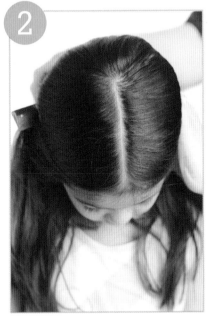

Using a tail comb, part the hair down the centre. Use her nose as the reference point for a perfect centre parting.

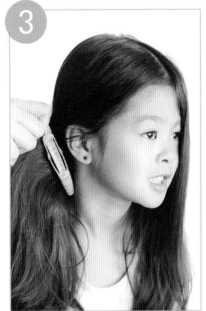

Clip one side out of the way so you can start to plait the other section.

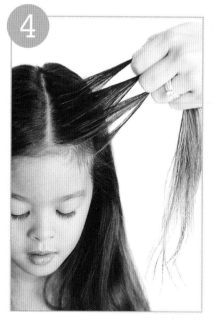

Starting at the top of the loose section, gather three pieces of hair.

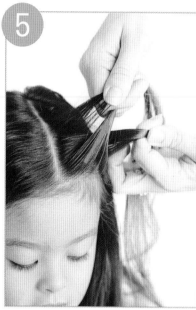

Cross the left section over the centre piece.

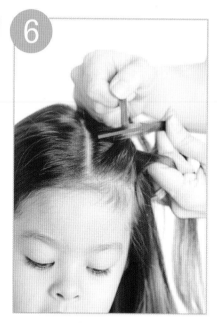

Next, cross the right section over the centre piece.

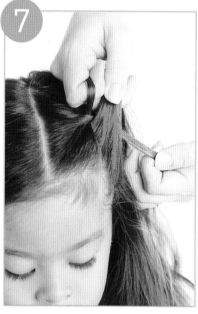

Grab a horizontal subsection of hair and add it to the left section. Cross your now larger left side over the centre piece.

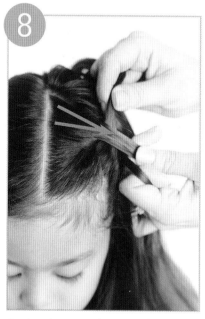

Grab a horizontal piece of hair and feed it into the right side section. Now cross that section over the centre section.

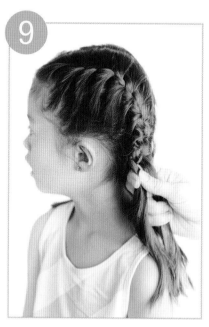

Continue with steps 7 and 8 until you reach the nape of her neck.

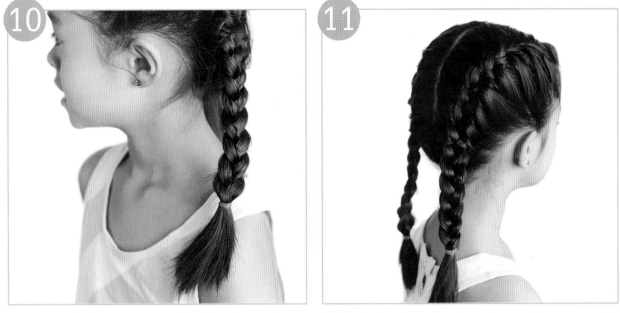

Continue to the bottom in a regular plait. Secure the ends with a colourful elastic.

Unclip the hair from the other side, and plait as you did on the first side.

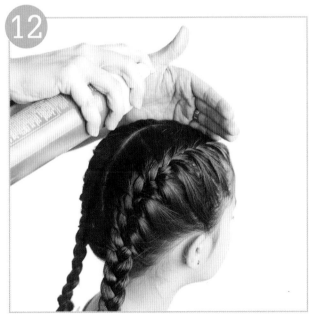

After you've secured the ends of the second plait, you can lightly spray with hairspray for extra hold.

Make waves

If you plait her hair while it's still wet, you can then unwind the plaits once they're dry to give her a head full of fun and funky waves.

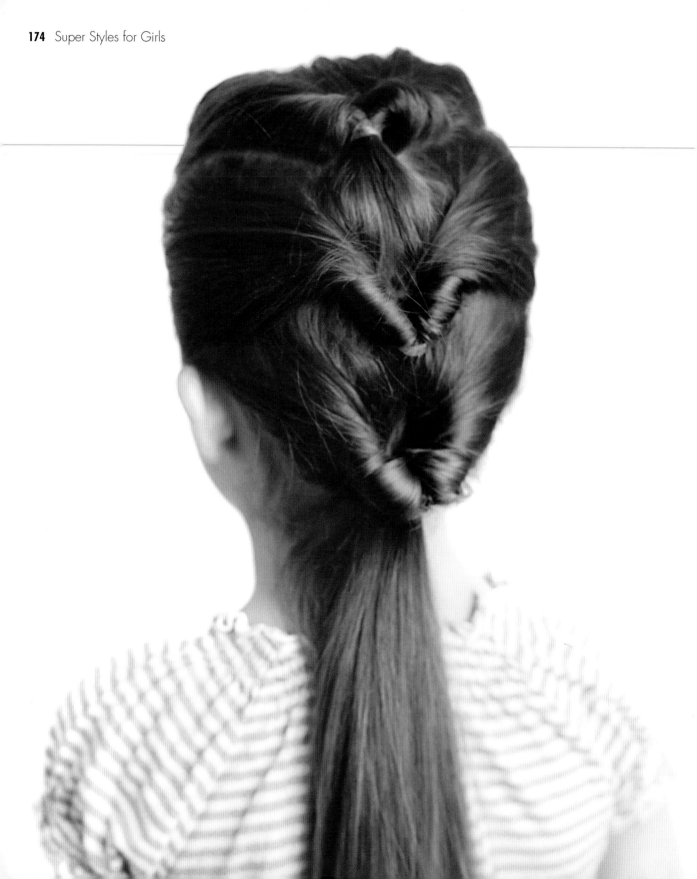

Twisted Sister

GIRLS

If you usually plait her hair using the basic plait, French plait or fishtail plait, this contemporary style will make a refreshing change. The Twisted Sister is a unique way to twist hair, but it's also highly practical. It may be attention-grabbing, but it's incredibly easy to create and will stand up to all sorts of activities.

Wavy and straight hair work best with this style. You can smooth a dollop of defining paste about 2cm in diameter into the hair at the start, before separating the hair out, for better grip. This also creates a more polished look for a special event.

TOOLS NEEDED

- colourful hair elastics
- hairspray
- tail comb

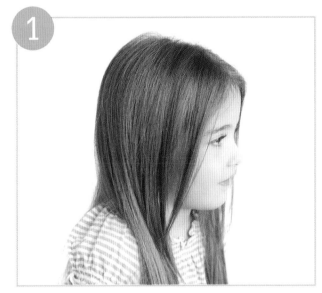

Start with dry hair that's been blow-dried smooth. It can have a slight wave in it, but not too much.

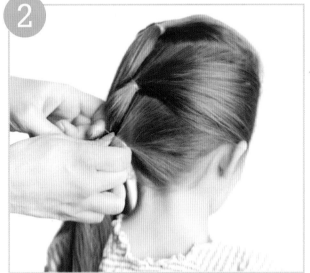

Using a tail comb, divide the hair into three equal horizontal sections. Secure each section with an elastic to give three separate ponytails, one on top of the other, down the back of the head.

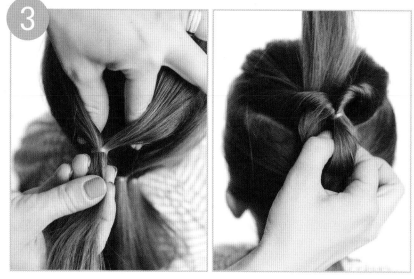
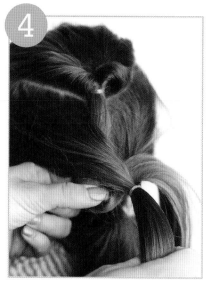

Turn the top ponytail inside out by creating a small hole directly above the first elastic and pulling the end of the tail through the opening.

Create an opening in the second ponytail (the middle one), and pull the tail of the top ponytail through the hole in the second.

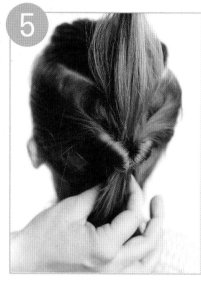
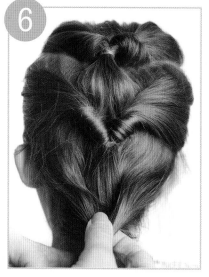
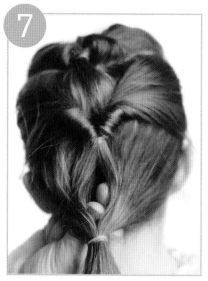

After you've pulled the tail through, create a new opening in the second ponytail just above the elastic, and pull the ponytail over and through the opening.

Make an opening just above the elastic in the third, bottom ponytail. Pull the tail from the second pony through the bottom opening. After you pull the ponytail through, you can use an additional elastic to secure it.

Create yet another opening directly above the elastic, and pull the end of the third ponytail over and into the opening, pulling the ponytail all the way through.

8

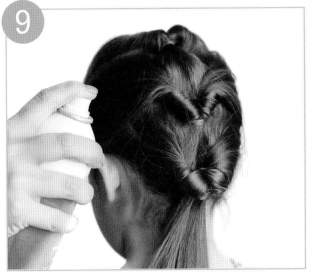

All three inside-out ponytails should be connected now.

9

Finish with hairspray for additional hold and to smooth hairs around the hairline

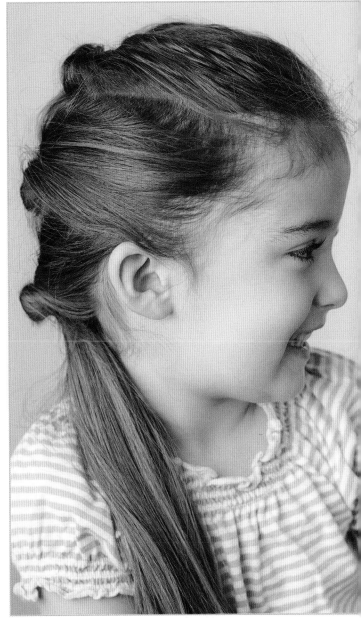

A little lift

For some additional volume, you can backcomb the crown slightly before separating into ponytails.

Glossary

ANTIFRIZZ SERUM This product tackles frizz by surrounding your hair strands with a protective, moisturizing coating. Depending on the type of serum, it can be used on wet or dry hair, and works well to combat frizz and tame unruly hair. In some cases, it can even reduce the amount of time your hair takes to dry.

ANTIHUMIDITY SERUM A styling product that blocks moisture, prevents frizz, and can help smooth your hair and tame flyaways.

ARGAN OIL This oil, produced from the kernels of a tree grown in Morocco, contains vitamins and essential fatty acids beneficial for your hair. It's great for times when your hair is damaged or needs moisture. As it absorbs into your hair, it hydrates and protects. It can be used on wet or dry locks.

BACKCOMBING BRUSH A brush, usually containing nylon and boar bristles, which is designed to add volume and texture to your hair.

BACKCOMBING COMB This is a comb with three rows of teeth and is used to backcomb your hair to increase volume. Don't use just any comb for backcombing; this special comb is vital for creating volume without damaging your hair.

BLOW-DRY A hairstyle created by applying a product to damp hair and then blow-drying the hair using a paddle brush and round brush for a voluminous effect. All lengths of hair can achieve this style in different variations.

BOAR BRISTLE BRUSH A brush that polishes your hair as you brush, thanks to the natural boar bristles, which help distribute your hair's natural oils.

BOB A short hairstyle; the length hits right at the jawline. The bob was especially popular in the 1920s.

BOBBY PIN See HAIR GRIP.

BRAID See PLAIT.

BUN SPONGE This styling aid helps you form the perfect bun. Using this doughnut-shape sponge, you pull your ponytail through the centre hole and then pin your hair around the doughnut to create a full, round bun. If you have trouble forming a voluminous bun with just your hair alone, try a bun sponge. They're available in a variety of colours and sizes.

CHIGNON A French word that means "nape of the neck". Also, a hairstyle in which a low-slung bun or knot sits close to the nape of the neck. These are usually worn in a formal setting and typically have a smooth and polished appearance.

CLEAR ELASTIC See HAIR ELASTIC.

CLIP Many sizes, shapes, and types of hair clips are available, but most often in this book, clip refers to a sturdy pinching clip with grips on one side to hold hair in place. You can find these clips at your beauty supply store.

CONCENTRATOR NOZZLE This fits on the end of a hairdryer and concentrates and directs air and heat flow, so you can dry your hair more smoothly. Using a concentrator nozzle on your hairdryer means you can get smoother and more polished hair without the use of straighteners.

CRIMPERS A heated tool that's designed to kink your hair into sharp, chevron or zigzag waves. This look was popular in the 1980s but has made a comeback on runways and at fancy-dress parties.

CROWN The top of the head. The hair in this area is easy to backcomb to create volume.

CURL CLIP This silver metal clip is approximately 5cm long and has two prongs. It's used to hold and set curls after they've been curled with tongs.

CURL CREAM This defines your curls and provides a light hold. You can layer curl cream with a light- or firm-hold gel for maximum hold. It is best applied to damp hair and then left to air dry or blow-dried using a diffuser.

CURLING IRON See CURLING TONGS.

CURLING TONGS This handheld tool has a barrel at one end that heats up. Multiple barrel sizes are available, ranging from 1cm to 5cm. You coil your hair around the hot barrel, close the clamp to keep your hair against the barrel, hold for a few seconds, and unclamp for curly locks. The larger the barrel, the bigger the curls.

CURLING WAND A handheld styling tool similar to curling tongs but without a clamp to hold your hair. This heated rod is great for getting mermaid waves.

DEFINING PASTE This is a lightweight finishing product that can be used to softly mould your hair. Applying a small amount throughout the hair adds texture to shorter hairstyles.

DIFFUSER NOZZLE This attachment fits on the end of your hairdryer and enhances curls by diffusing the air and heat widely and evenly. It also helps to reduce frizz when drying curly hair.

DRY SHAMPOO This a quick-and-easy way to extend your style over several days. It asborbs oil and freshens up any type of hair. You also can add texture to your hair by applying dry shampoo to your roots before backcombing. This is great for formal styles as well.

ELASTIC See HAIR ELASTIC.

FIRM-HOLD GEL This gel is able to set your hair with maximum hold. Formal styles and up-dos that require extra hold can benefit from this product before blow-drying to ensure the style lasts all night. You can also help control stubborn curls using a firm-hold gel.

FISHTAIL PLAIT A variation of a plait that's woven to look like a fishbone.

FLAT IRON See STRAIGHTENERS

FRENCH PLAIT A plait that starts at the top of the head and is woven downwards to the very ends of the hair.

FRINGE The area typically from the edge of one eyebrow to the other on the front hairline.

HAIR ELASTIC The clear version of these elastic bands, usually 1cm to 2cm in diameter, are commonly used in up-styles and formal hairdos, since they're not easily visible in the finished style. Coloured elastics are also available, either to match your hair colour, or to add a pop of bright colour to a ponytail or the end of a plait.

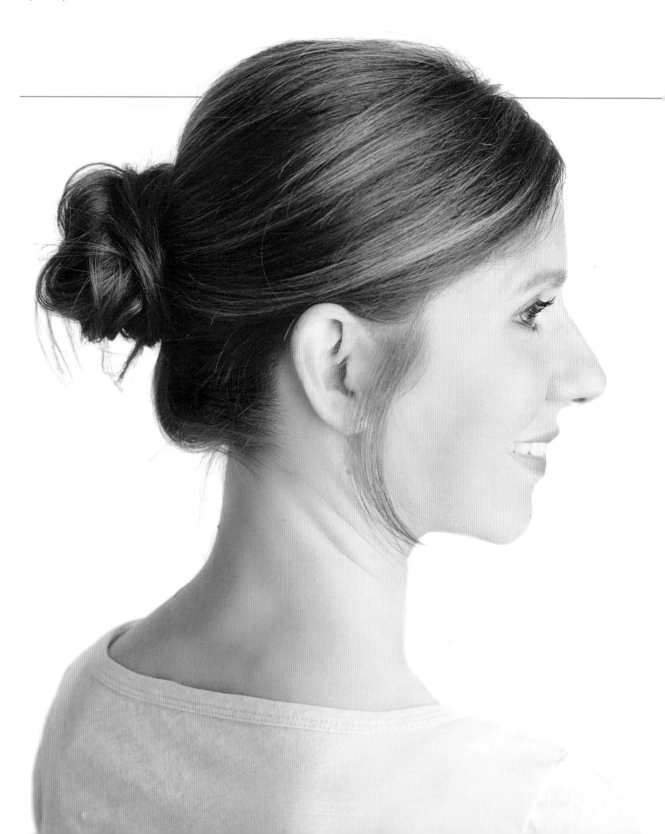

HAIR GRIP These small, wavy pins hold hair firmly in place, making them an essential part of any up-do style. Standard grips are about 5cm long, but you can also get smaller and larger sizes. They come in a variety of colours to blend in with your hair.

HAIRPIN A U-shape pin that secures your hair without disrupting the flow of your hairstyle. Whereas a hair grip offers firm hold, hairpins have a very loose and natural hold. They come in various lengths and colours.

HAIRLINE The area where your hair meets your skin.

HAIR POWDER See VOLUMIZING POWDER.

HEAT-RESISTANT COMB A comb that can stand up to the heat produced by hot tools and won't melt. You can use it to guide and keep your hair smooth while you use curling tongs or straighteners. A good general comb can also be used to coax hair into up-dos.

HOT ROLLERS Cylindrical curling tools that heat up in an electric device. When they're hot, you wind your hair around them and clip them into place to set. When they're cool, you remove them to release the curls.

HYDRATING CONDITIONER Curly hair, or any hair prone to frizz, should choose a hydrating conditioner. It's especially useful in the winter months when the dry air caused by central heating can cause static.

HYDRATING SHAMPOO This shampoo is designed for dry or dull hair. If you have fine hair, you'll most likely want to avoid hydrating or moisturizing shampoos, which can weigh your hair down. Medium to thick and coarse hair types benefit most from this shampoo.

HEAT PROTECTOR A spray or cream that helps protect your hair from heated styling tools. Typically these are used on dry hair; you can use some on wet or damp hair as well.

KIRBY GRIP See Hair Grip.

LEAVE-IN CONDITIONER This comes as either a cream or a spray. Most leave-in treatments contain a moisture-retention ingredient and offer differing amounts of moisture to suit different hair types. Many also give your hair extra shine.

MAXIMUM-HOLD HAIRSPRAY This hairspray usually includes an antihumidity ingredient that protects your hair against the environment and prolongs your style. Max-hold sprays are typically used in formal styles.

MOISTURIZING SERUM This product is used to soften and relax hair. Argan oil, antifrizz serums, or any kind of serum that contains moisturizing ingredients are all moisturizing serums.

MOULDING PASTE See DEFINING PASTE.

MOUSSE Also known as styling foam, this multitasking product is used to add volume to your roots and the ends of your hair while also providing a light hold. It tames and helps shape your hair but doesn't leave it brittle and dry.

PADDLE BRUSH This large, flat brush is used to detangle and speed up drying time when blow-drying. The soft bristles are designed to be gentle on wet or dry hair.

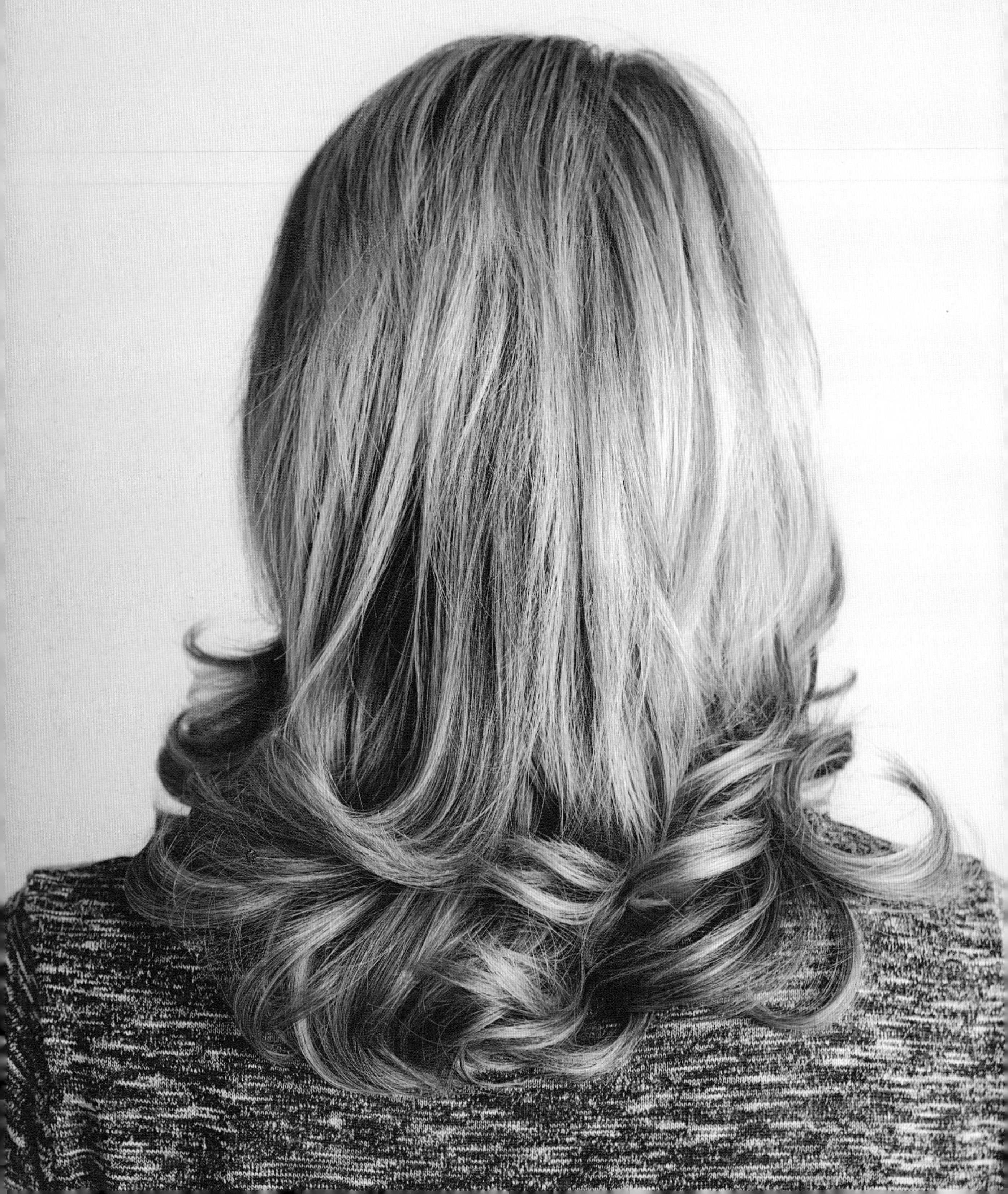

PARTING A division in your hair. You create a parting by drawing a line on your scalp with a comb or your fingers.

POMADE This is a light-hold finishing product that defines your strands and adds polish and shine.

REPAIRING CONDITIONER This product often contains a type of protein or keratin treatment to help strengthen weak or damaged hair. It's a good idea to use a repairing conditioner on a weekly basis if you regularly colour your hair or use heated tools.

REPAIRING SHAMPOO This shampoo is designed to improve the look and feel of damaged hair, and helps prevent future breakage.

ROLLERS See HOT ROLLERS.

ROLY POLY See BUN SPONGE

ROOT The part of your hair that emerges from your scalp.

ROOT LIFTER A root booster or lifter helps lift your hair from the roots in your crown area.

ROUND BRUSH This brush is essential for smoothing, taming, and curling your hair. Some are vented or have a ceramic barrel to speed up drying. Many sizes are available: a smaller round brush produces a curly or wavier look in the middle and at the ends of your hair, whereas a larger size mainly smooths your hair and gives a slight bend at the ends.

SCULPTING LOTION This light-hold liquid gives hair hold without adding weight. It's best used before you curl your hair or to add longevity to your style.

SEA-SALT SPRAY Usually sprayed on the ends of damp hair, this helps promote a natural, beach-wave look. Those with wavy or curly hair to start with can achieve soft waves with this mist; straight hair will gain texture and a touch of bend.

SECTIONING CLIP This long, flat clip ranges from 5cm to 10cm long. As well as sectioning off hair while styling, it is often used to hold curls, as it doesn't leave creases like a curl clip does.

SHINE SPRAY Used mostly as a finishing product, this mist is designed to enhance shine and bring life to dull-looking hair.

SMOOTHING SERUM This product typically contains an antifrizz or antihumidity property to coax wavy, coarse, or curly hair smooth and straight, and add moisture. Many contain ingredients that help protect against future damage.

SPLIT ENDS A condition in which the ends of your strands of hair are literally split in two. This is a sign that your hair has been damaged and is in need of a trim.

SPRAY WATER BOTTLE Use this to wet your hair when you need moisture during a style. You can find them at your local chemist.

SPRAY WAX This liquid wax has a light to medium hold designed to bring texture to the hair. Fine to medium hair types will benefit most from its thickening effect.

STRAIGHTENERS A handheld tool that uses heat to style your hair, straighteners (or straightening irons) have two ceramic plates that close together, sandwiching your hair in between, to smooth and flatten your hair. Flat irons can get extremely hot, reaching temperatures upwards of 200°C.

STYLING FOAM See MOUSSE.

TAIL COMB This comb has small teeth on one end and a straight, pointy pick on the other end. The pointy end is helpful for precisely sectioning and parting your hair before styling.

TEXTURE PUTTY This putty gives you a strong yet workable hold. Texture putty works best for shaping shorter styles. Many are transparent but if the putty is light in colour, it's best to use it on lighter-coloured hair.

TEXTURIZING SPRAY A styling product that adds more movement or grit to your original hair texture. Spray wax or sea-salt spray are examples.

THERMAL PROTECTANT See HEAT PROTECTOR.

THICKENING CONDITIONER This is for use alongside thickening shampoo. It adds extra volume to limp or lifeless stands. It also softens your strands without weighing them down.

THICKENING LOTION Designed to coat each of your strands to make them fuller, thickening lotion is best for very fine hair that needs more body. It can be used as a light-hold product as well.

THICKENING SHAMPOO This shampoo is best for those whose hair is thinning or who have very fine hair to begin with. It often contains an exfoliating ingredient to unclog follicles and give your strands the best possible chance of growth, as well as thickness boosting ingredients.

THREE-BARREL CURLING TONGS Curling tongs with multiple barrels – typically two on the bottom and one on the top. Pressing your hair between the barrels creates soft, uniform waves.

VENT BRUSH A brush with slots in the body of the brush, between the bristles. When you blow-dry your hair, air flows through, allowing it to dry faster.

VOLUMIZING CONDITIONER This can be used to soften your tresses and doesn't leave behind any residue. A lightweight volumizing conditioner benefits fine to medium hair types.

VOLUMIZING HAIRSPRAY A hairspray that promotes volume with a firm hold.

VOLUMIZING POWDER This is applied to the roots of dry hair for added fullness. Some types of hair powder will reactivate throughout the day with a little massage from your fingers. This powder provides a tousled, voluminous look.

VOLUMIZING SHAMPOO This lightweight shampoo gives limp locks some volume. It's usually colourless and should give your hair a weightless feel.

WIDE-TOOTH COMB The teeth on this comb are spaced a bit wider apart than on other types of combs. This helps you gently work through tangles and is especially good on wet hair.

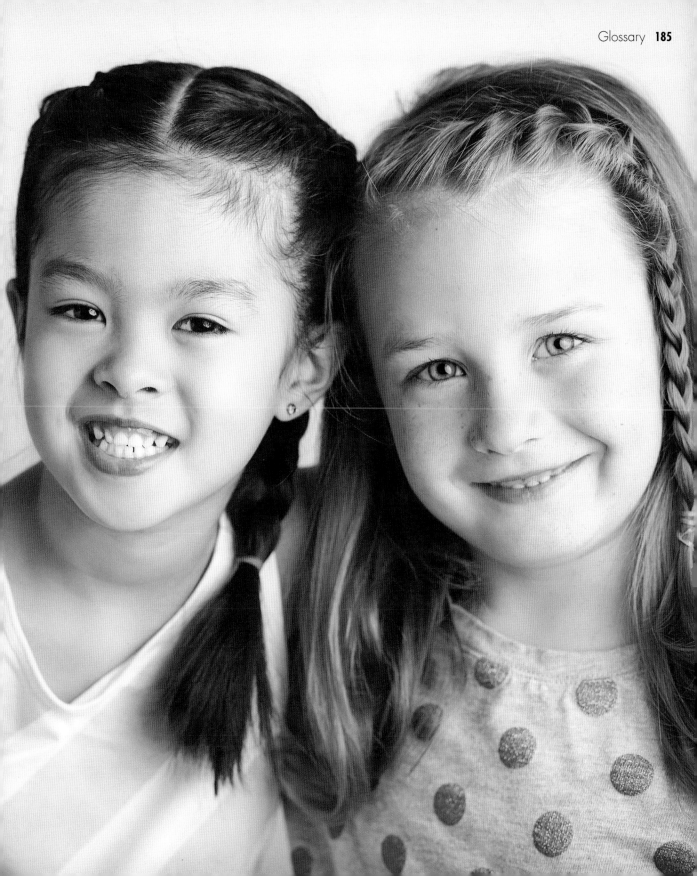

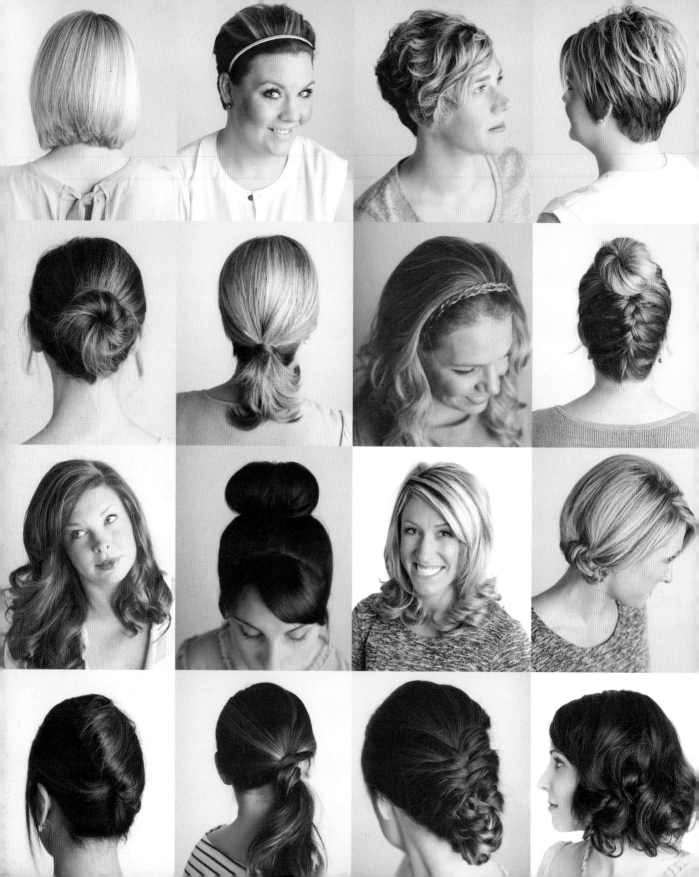

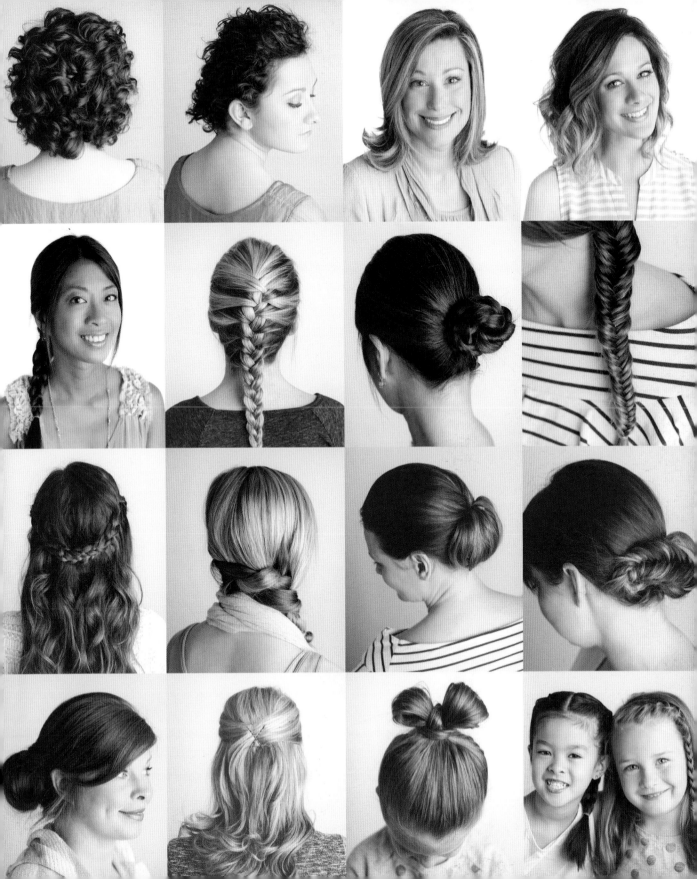

Index

Publisher's Acknowledgments

Dorling Kindersley would like to thank Era Chawla, Navidita Thapa, and Bushra Ahmed in the India Delhi office and Kathryn Meeker and Glenda Fisher in the UK London office. Also, Kate Berens for Alglicising the British edition. For photo credits, Dorling Kindersley would like to thank Heather Hughes for the top image on the front jacket (hair brush and combs).

Author's Acknowledgments

I'd like to extend an enormous thank you to my team at Alpha Books for all their enthusiasm, hard work, and help making this book as fabulous as it can possibly be: my editor Christy Wagner, book designer/photographer Becky Batchelor, and managing editor Billy Fields. Thanks to Christie Wright and Mary Landwer for their helpful assistance in making the hairstyles come to life. Also, thanks to Tess Payton for her mad make-up skills and making our models look their personal best. Thank you to all the beautiful models – Alicia Mummert, Brittany Case, Carly Grant, Christie Wright, Heather Stafford, Jenni Davis, Jessica Kelly, Josie Sanders, Jourdyn Berry, Julie and Kennedy Williams, Kirsten Becker, Kristi and Mia Johnson, Marian Bender, Mary Landwer, Monica Johnson, Mya Fields, Shelby Dock, and Sophia Batchelor – for taking time out of your busy schedules to help create the images for this book. Next, I owe an enormous amount of gratitude to my husband, Ryan, for holding down the fort while I was hard at work trying to make this book come to life, but most of all for always believing in me. My friends and family – you all know who you are. It's a great comfort to know that I have an awesome support system and that you all have cheered me on throughout this incredible journey, especially Ronny Douglas, Judy Bond, and Christy Rushton. As they say, "it takes a village", and I have an amazing one behind me. A huge thanks to my mother, Marcia, for encouraging me to always do my best and believing I could truly do whatever I set my heart on. In addition, thank you to my clients and the readers of this book for allowing me to live my dream as a professional hairstylist. I appreciate each and every one of you and realize this all would not be possible without you. It's truly an honour to be able to make people look and feel their best.

ABOUT THE AUTHOR

Kylee Bond is the co-owner of and hair stylist at Kindred: A Beauty Lounge (kindredbeautylounge.com). After earning her Bachelors in Managements at The University of New Orleans, USA, Kylee graduated from the Aveda Frederic's Institute. A few years of hands-on experience and valuable industry knowledge, coupled with hard work, enabled Kylee to open her first award-winning salon. Kylee's passion shows through her work as she creates the perfect cut, colour, and style for each of her clients.

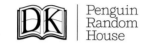

TEAM FOR ALPHA BOOKS
Publisher Mike Sanders
Executive Managing Editor Billy Fields
Development Editorial Supervisor Christy Wagner
Senior Designer Becky Batchelor
Senior Production Editor Janette Lynn
Indexer Johnna VanHoose Dinse
Proofreader Monica Stone
Photography Becky Batchelor Photography

TEAM FOR DK
Project Editor Claire Cross
Senior Designer Anne Fisher
Managing Editor Stephanie Farrow
Managing Art Editor Christine Keilty

First published by Penguin Group (USA) Inc. in 2014

This edition published in 2016 by
Dorling Kindersley Limited,
80 Strand, London WC2R 0RL

A CIP catalogue record for this book
is available from the British Library.
ISBN 978-0-2412-3726-7

Printed and bound in China.

All images © Dorling Kindersley Limited
For further information see: www.dkimages.com

A WORLD OF IDEAS:
SEE ALL THERE IS TO KNOW

www.dk.com